Pr

Humanity's Cry for Change

I choose to see the bright side of this amazing planet. With all my training and reading, I could not get to the light with the shutdown of my chiropractic business due to COVID-19. And then…an amazing intervention by God, The Creator, as Kate calls this beautiful force of light and love, started to shine on me. Kate asked me to read and review her second book.

This book reminded me that we're all in this together. Kate beautifully points out the tremendous opportunity that awaits: a global healing, a reckoning to shift universal consciousness and raise humankind to the next level of enlightenment. She thoughtfully explains the process. She specifically gives exercises and strategies and most important, her book shifted me from fear to love.

The Universe has always had impeccable timing. Kate's book is on point to shift humanity towards love, light and compassion. Everyone should read this book.

— Dr. Greg Mortimer, DC

I love this book! It is a timely reflection on how to transform the chaotic world we are living in to a world filled with more joy, compassion, peace and harmony. Kate Heartsong is an inspirational author, and I loved the effective exercises she has in this book. The book provides hope in a world that can sometimes leave us feeling hopeless and helpless. A must read!

— Dot Kaufman

I consider myself a seasoned reader of self-help books, so I was completely taken by surprise that here in these pages were really refreshing and important NEW information. Kate Heartsong includes a roadmap and compass on how we are going to finally get to the new way of being we all long for. Inspiring, with 'feet on the ground' step-by-step practicality—Kate is on the level of Joan Borysenko and Marianne Williamson. I will read this book again and again. Thank you, Kate, for being the conduit we all desperately need in this time of accelerated change. Namaste.

— Susan Parchman

Kate Heartsong gives a wide variety of comfortable exercises that fit a variety of personal needs. She has an amazing ability to demonstrate easy ways we each effectuate changes in ourselves and in the lives of others. She brings forth so beautifully how and why we are truly all interconnected, and why it is time to reconsider that I have the individual power to make change every day. This book gives me tangible daily activities I can incorporate easily into my day or my week toward a goal of improving how I feel, and that I can positively affect how other beings on our planet feel also! This is a must read for the times we are in and I am fortunate to have received these wonderful insights.

— Elionore Gruber

This book is a brilliant account of the vibrational shift that is taking place on our planet today and the desperate need for change on an individual and global basis. The author explores a new awareness of Oneness that shifts our consciousness from head to heart-felt living which has the potential to raise our vibrational levels. She shares powerful insights, knowledge and tools on how to heal ourselves and our planet and gives hope to the possibility that we can change. This is a transformational book with powerful insights and tools that is timely and truly needed in these times!

— Angela Casola Ph.D. Professor at Metro State University

A beautifully written book filled with love and possibilities for a more harmonious future. My heart expanded when I read this book. Easy to follow exercises to help you align with who you truly are. A Gift.   — Vicky Golder

I found that *Humanity's Cry for Change* provides a vast array of important insights as well as practical exercises to help anyone navigate through the evolving changes influencing our planet. In an easy to follow manner, Kate empowers the reader to know that individuals will—through our natural influence of consciousness—make positive differences for ourselves, our communities and the planet. She even shares key points in which the business community can support sustainability and optimal outcomes.

Kate shows why it's important to understand how we are all interconnected, and gives some scientific evidence that supports this principle. I highly recommend reading this book if you want effective guidance to navigate through the current planetary and individual shifts that we are all experiencing!

— Rich Haas, author of *Sacred Quantum Metaphysics*

Kate Heartsong's book offers a mindful viewpoint to explain earth's current evolution. She explores the many changes that are already taking place individually, locally, globally and even corporately, both the good and bad. Kate provides an abundance of examples, relatable analogies and exercises. In this very busy world, regularly using techniques like the self-exploration and inner guidance will help me to be my most authentic self. All the tools she provides can be used to help affect positive personal growth and in doing so, influence others and our sacred earth for the better.   — Liz Cooksey

Humanity's Cry for Change is an insightful and timely guide for humans finding themselves in the middle of a great change. Ms. Heartsong takes a careful look at what is needed to achieve a new level of understanding of ourselves and a higher quality of life. Ms. Heartsong thoroughly discusses the challenges and offers a means for individuals to change their own perspectives, to heal their hearts and to change their consciousness. The exercises, offered in step by step guidance, are concrete and in varied ways for individuals to heal and transcend ego-based living. For those who are ready to connect at a communal level, the discussion in

Section Four is specific and helpful. Thank you, Ms. Heartsong. Well Done! — J. Tomas

Kate explains what is happening in the old Earth paradigm so clearly that we cannot help but see why many of us have felt so uncomfortable for so long trying to live in a system that is out of alignment. Lightworkers came here to create the new Earth and we have been shining the best we could in the old system, but Kate helps us see now how to shine our way TO the new world we are each playing our part in creating together. If you are seeking your way in this time of transition, this is the book for you to read now.

— Tracy Maxwell, author of *Being Single, With Cancer*. Founder of HazingPrevention.Org

I love this book! Throughout I receive the loving voice of the author, Kate Heartsong. There is no doubt that what brought Kate to write this book is her deep and compassionate concern for Mother Earth and Humanity. Skillfully, with strokes of her pen, Kate paints a firm and clear picture of the situation our world faces right now.

Her easy to do and uplifting exercises is the answer to our dilemma. These present the reader with an alternative to following the status quo. In them, the reader is shown that setting intention towards self-awareness and improvement, each one of us can make a difference in moving the needle to positive social and environmental change. I especially resonated with the exercises that emphasize living in the present moment. In addition, the exercises that direct the reader to notice, enjoy and harness the chi energy within and around us, were powerful and cogent. The entire book leaves me feeling calm and peaceful! Kate left me, as it will leave the reader, with hope for our future.

— Linda Stopp, MPA

Prayer for the New Earth

May we come to know
The vibrancy and delight
Of our authentic selves
Fulfilling our true destiny

May the light of our love
Shine in our eyes
Looking upon all creation
Knowing we are all one united

May we know in our hearts
True inner peace and joy
Radiating this out as kindness and laughter
To all our brothers and sisters

May we honor and respect
Our dear Mother Earth
For the abundance she shares so freely
Sustaining our bodies, hearts and souls

May we come to know
In our lifetime the experience of
The love, peace and joy of the new earth
That is the birthright of humanity

— Kate Heartsong

HUMANITY'S CRY FOR
Change

Actions You
Can Take to Create
a New Earth

Kate Heartsong

Humanity's Cry for Change
Actions You Can Take to Create a New Earth
by Kate Heartsong

Published by

Joyful Radiance Company, LLC
Lakewood, Colorado

ISBN: 978-0-9842492-3-7 (print)
Library of Congress Control Number: 2020906047

BISAC Category: Philosophy/movements; Inspirational/personal growth; Self-help/motivational

Cover design by Natasha S. Brown
Interior design by NZ Graphics
Editing by The Red Pen Editor

Quantity purchase: Contact the author at www.JoyfulRadiance.com

First Edition

Printed in the United State of America

This book is dedicated to
humanity
and
to all lightworkers and awakened ones

Contents

Introduction

G reat paradigm shifts and changes in the way humanity approaches life occurs at certain times throughout all of humanity's history. The most monumental paradigm shift of all of mankind's history is happening now. You are likely aware of the heightened anxiety and fluctuating emotions over global virus pandemics, the increase in global violence, financial meltdowns, worldwide economic crisis, the rise in the number of natural disasters, increased terrorism, the climate crises, and lack of respect for Mother Earth and her people.

You have likely heard about grassroot movements, such as Occupy Wallstreet, movements for climate change, and various other types of organizations that are bringing into your awareness the alarming harmful activities taking place on our planet. It is vital we become aware of these so we can act to reduce or eliminate these negative activities and their effects. For example, genetically modified organisms (GMOs) are becoming more widespread and many people worldwide are unhealthy as a result. Many organizations are bringing pressure and offering education to people to thwart off the overtaking by certain large companies who have an invested interest (money and power) to perpetuate the GMOs.

All of these, plus many more, are demonstrations of the upheavals in what you know as the current paradigm existing on our planet. These upheavals are a necessary change that comes with the shift of our current state of affairs and its associated transition from a male dominated, competitive, capitalized era with an emphasis on mental intelligence, to what is necessary to save humanity—a "new earth"— represented by an era that has a more equal balance between men and women, a respect and understanding of the diversity of people on the planet, and for Mother Earth herself, a dominance of collaboration and sharing of resources, giving equality and equity to everyone, a perspective of living life knowing all life is interconnected, and improved social enterprise including treating all workers with respect and fairness.

This current and new evolutionary leap includes the innate changes that are happening with Mother Earth, for she, too, is undergoing the evolutionary shift. It is law, just as gravity is a law. It simply takes place and you are in the very midst of the most precedented shift of all of humanity: The Age of Aquarius. This major shift occurs every 26,000 years. You can reference Gregg Braden's book *Fractal Time* for more in-depth details of this 26,000-year cycle that is now transitioning into a new 26,000-year cycle. The Mayan's calendar ended on December 21, 2012, not to predict the world ending but rather to indicate the end of the 26,000-year cycle and the beginning of a new 26,000-year cycle.

With the beginning of every new cycle and subsequent shift, whether it is planetary wide or individually, a dismantling of the old paradigm occurs. This is indeed a birthing process and this process requires the releasing of the old, in order to make room for the new! Humanity is in the very midst of this monumental shift.

In order to reach the new earth more effectively and easily, several actions must take place:

- Each individual will do best to flow and change with the predominate shift happening worldwide. Those who resist this shift, both vibrationally and physically, have a harder time adapting to the newer environment.

- Each person will adapt easier to this shift when they live from higher vibrational emotions such as love, kindness and respect, versus the sharp contrast to those with lower vibrational emotions such as anger, jealousy or hatred.

- Each person will optimize living their life experience by living authentically and in alignment with their true essence. This means to genuinely live in such a way that honors your true character and nature, and to offer your real gifts and talents.

- On an organizational, community, or enterprise level, what is required to effectively bring in the new earth requires considering all components of a system that are affected when creating a new organization, business, construction project or community organization. It also requires successfully implementing policies and procedures to support equity for, and inclusion of, the diverse employees as well as the clients or customers of any organization.

When every person offers their important piece of the whole puzzle, then the whole puzzle is nicely filled in and this creates a fluidity that carries the whole of humanity in a synergistic proper balance. It is this synergistic balance that facilitates, on a global level, a higher vibration of love, and naturally leads to a planet of peace.

Imagine with me what it would be like to use Mother Earth's resources in a capacity that supports optimal usage of resources, resulting in all people having enough food to eat.

See the world where strangers are generous and kind to others, knowing there are plenty of resources available to go around, whether it is food, gas, water, or money.

Think about a world in which your children feel and *are* safe to walk any street in the world, because there is only the kindness and respect offered to each person throughout the world.

Feel what it would personally be like if you were in a position to relax and be stress free, to be working in a field or career that truly makes your heart sing.

What would you feel like if you had no worries about where your next meal or money for rent came from?

What would your grandchildren's future look like if you knew there will always be truth and honesty offered by all people?

Imagine what the world would look like, and be like, if all people *knew and lived* with the knowing that *all* people are indeed created equal, and that no one person, that no one religion, that no one country, that no one type of skin color, that no one type of life style, is better than another.

This sounds like utopia, yes? Indeed, it can be described as just this!

And, it is possible.

You see, with this evolutionary shift, the evolutionary shift of higher consciousness, people and Mother Earth's vibration is rising. It is this rising in vibration that represents a rising into love, a rising into a better *capacity and ability* to actually live from this place of higher respect, kindness and love for one's self and for all. For it is these ingredients called The Creator's qualities that facilitates, empowers, and puts into motion the very utopia just described. For without the ability or capacity to be in the higher vibrations (love, gratitude, respect, kindness and so on), the violence and war will continue. The lower vibrations (hate, jealousy, anger, violence, greed and so on) cannot be sustained for much longer, for the nature of this 26,000-year evolutionary shift is the rising of consciousness, and inherent in this— the very law of this—is such that the old, lower vibrations are being eliminated and released, so that the new higher vibrations can enter and be upheld in a better fashion.

And since this evolutionary leap is occurring, why not make it easier on yourself by taking on the exercises in this book that will help make this birthing process easier for you? Would you not also want this for your children and your children's children?

In order to understand and become more aware with greater insight, there are certain principles and teachings that will assist you in understanding why the planet is currently experiencing the huge upheavals of terrorism, war, and violence; why there is an increase in self-hatred, which is projected onto others; why there is a sharp increase in the number of school shootings and domestic violence; and why there is less respect for Mother Earth and her resources.

Through this understanding and insight, you will then have a better desire and be more motivated to make change in your personal life because you will realize *it starts with you.* For you are the only person that can make change in your life. When enough people do this, it affects the collective consciousness, and this then creates the pivotal breaking point where then more and more people become awake and live in the higher vibrational emotions such as love and gratitude that are needed.

"You have always had the power, my dear," said Glinda the good witch to Dorothy in the movie *The Wizard of Oz.* So, come on this insightful journey to discover how to change, not only your life, but to change humanity and the planet. When many of us take action for change, the whole planet shifts and peace can again reign on Mother Earth, reign in your heart and your life, reign in the lives of those you love, and reign for the future generations of humanity.

You will receive hope by reading this book. You will see, that starting with you, it *is* possible to make a positive difference in your life. This book will also share some vital insights by which life can be lived to better propagate and facilitate the *natural* way of living; living from the perspective of Oneness—Oneness Living—the understanding that all of life is interconnected. This results in making a positive difference to you, to those around you, and to the whole planet.

Throughout this book you will read the term "The Creator," which references what some may know as The Universe, Lord, Father, Source, The One, God, or The I Am. Certainly, replace the term with whichever term resonates with you.

Peace within, peace on earth.

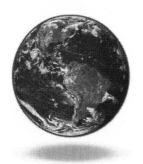

SECTION 1

What on Earth is Happening?

Optimal Living

Two hundred thousand years ago, and for thousands of years after, people lived with the understanding that there is an interconnectivity between all life. This was the *way* of life. Not knowing any other way of living, there was a great respect and honoring toward all life, of how life flowed, of how to interact optimally with Mother Earth and her resources and with others. This understanding was passed from one generation to the next.

The benefit of living from this interconnected perspective is that of widespread respect and consideration for *all* life and also for all individual components of a system, such as farming, where land use is rotated every few years. Also, this helps to understand that what a person does to another, they do to themselves. In the beginning of humanity, the understanding of Oneness Living, that is, the interconnection of all life, was the normal way to live. This approach supports living in an easier and more efficient manner and also encourages honoring *all* components of a system.

There have been a number of upgrades in humanity's intellect as its consciousness gradually evolved over time, starting about 10,000 years ago. Consequently, there was a shift from living with the understanding that all life is interconnected, to living more from believing we are separate from other people, from animals, and from Mother Earth, resulting in an increased focus on living more for ourselves rather than considering everyone involved in any given situation or group.

When there is an emphasis on living from this individualistic perspective, there is an increase in competition, aggression, masculine energy being out of balance with feminine energy, and an increased level of disrespect for all aspects of the whole. A new way of life was created over each era of humanity, gradually starting about 10,000 years ago to the present time, in which more and more emphasis was placed on modernization and an evolutionary leap occurred once again. The collective consciousness of humanity changes over time as the perceptions of more and more people change over time.

Now the time has come to stop the current dominance of the left-brain intellect and masculine energies. This focus of masculine energies has resulted in the disharmony, grievances, difficulties, and wars on the planet. Although there is no right or wrong with how the orientation or perspective is for humanity, there is an *optimal* way of approaching life. This optimal way is to understand and live from the perspective that *all* life is interconnected. Humanity is being encouraged to cultivate and propagate once again the knowing that there is a unity and connection with all life, whereby enabling greater respect and kindness to all, including Mother Earth. This in turn can support creating an era of peace and harmony. For without this shift away from the masculine energies, competitiveness, disrespect, a separation perspective and imbalance, the destruction of all life on planet earth is inevitable.

This is why it is *imperative* that humans come back to what was the norm of living 200,000 years ago: the awareness of and living by the concept of Oneness Living. Without going back to the roots of realizing and living from this unity perspective, there will be continued destruction on our planet.

But make no mistake about it, there is, and always has been, a natural tendency for life to balance itself to the proper homeostasis. It is in this proper homeostasis environment in which the natural order of life is restored. Through this natural balancing, there will, once again, be peace on our planet. This will be more in alignment with the way life is *meant* to be lived, that is, in an *optimized* fashion.

There are those among humanity that exemplify and demonstrate this natural way of living. These people are what some refer to as lightworkers, and can also be called those who are awake. The characteristics found among most lightworkers include high vibrational frequencies of love, respect, understanding, reverence for *all* life, working in harmony with Mother Earth and *all* its creatures, peaceful living, a healthy respect for how to treat all of life, a *natural* way of healing disease, having healthy relationships with a foundation of unconditional love, and acceptance of *all* people. In short, all the qualities of The Creator.

Living in this way optimizes the whole of the ecosystem called Mother Earth, along with her human, plant, and animal inhabitants that she is assigned to take care of. When humans disregard Mother Earth's resources, the very resources that facilitate her inhabitant's lives, her ability to take care of her inhabitants becomes compromised. The resulting difficulties of living are the natural consequences that occur. For example, due to humanity's misuse of Mother Earth's natural resources, there is gross misalignment and imbalance in many areas on the planet, causing world hunger. And, with the continual raping of Mother Earth's resources, it is difficult to provide necessary water to many regions of the planet.

All of these can, and must, be resolved to restore Mother Earth's ability to provide for her inhabitants. Without the necessary changes of respecting and properly interacting with Mother Earth, there will be nothing left to sustain her inhabitants.

The current movement of sustainability is moving humanity toward the right direction of increased respect and proper usage of Mother Earth's gifts. Sustainability offers complete regard and respect for how living organisms, such as fish or plants, interact naturally with each other and with the environment in which they live. Permaculture is a prime example of this. Permaculture encompasses all the necessary components that optimize the use of all the individual elements, which allows further propagation and encourages a more integrated synergistic entity.

More community-like groups are necessary to optimize the resources of our Mother Earth in a way that then facilitates a better use of resources overall. This in turn cultivates and supplies enough food and water resources for all the people in their community. It is using the natural energy that is already there, which then produces an outcome that optimally provides resources when initiating the food-providing system.

In the same way, when there is a thorough understanding of the way nature normally is, then you can best optimize the individual components to produce the most natural outcome you are intending to get. There are components that can and need to be used in a certain proportion so the outcome of, say a process or system, is optimized. *And herein lies the crux of this writing:* when all projects, groups, and efforts understand the assimilations of the required components, the intricacies of the interactions with all those components, and the interconnectedness of all the required components, the outcome will be optimized. This is best accomplished by respecting all of the necessary components and realizing the effect that one has on another, similar to the domino effect. Some natural outcomes affect those components (say, the river or the wildlife) in certain ways and through these effects, the whole is influenced.

There are many processes going on throughout the planet, and when pooled together, there is a great impact on the whole planet. There is an incongruence within so many processes, and this has caused an imbalance within the arena where the processes are occurring. To have a process work optimally, it is best to approach creating and maintaining the process from a sustainable, wholistic, unified, respectful, and loving manner. This is what is required to bring all of life into a more optimal way of being, which naturally leads to a higher vibration. When life can have more of this higher vibration, then what can occur is increased alignment, unison, and optimization of Mother Earth's resources.

And it is this increased alignment, unison, and optimization of Mother Earth's resources we are striving to increase. More education as well as open mindedness and a shift and a change of heart are required to support making this change. The understanding of how components, processes and systems affect the whole and thoughtfulness of how they impact the whole are necessary for taking effective action.

It is time to shift into the consciousness of Oneness Living, sustainability, awareness of our actions and its impact on the whole, and to offer respect for *all* individual components of the whole. Through this, there is a far greater opportunity to create living in an optimal way across all forms of life.

Alignment with Mother Earth

As previously stated, humanity is going through a new evolutionary phase. This is a leap into a new age of humanity known as the Age of Aquarius. In all evolutionary phases there are growing pains caused by changes in the paradigm. Change is not always easy; however, change is necessary.

There are many changes happening on our planet. Mother Earth goes through evolutionary leaps as well for she is a living organism, no different than any other life form. There are many areas of growth, regeneration, shifts, expansion, and changes inherent in a living organism such as Mother Earth. Due to all of life having interconnection, humans go through the growing pains that Mother Earth goes through. For most, this is felt unconsciously by the masses, and for some, on a conscious level. When we can be in more harmony and respect with Mother Earth's changes, we as a species can flow easier with life, be in more harmony and have improved sustainability. We can reap the bounty of Mother Earth's gifts in a more efficient way when we live in proper alignment.

What do we mean by proper alignment? It is living with and from the land with reverence and with respect. When a person lives from this perspective and orientation, then a lifestyle naturally comes that is conducive to reaping Mother

Earth's benefits in an efficient and optimal manner. It is from this efficient and optimal manner that allows *all* of Mother Earth's inhabitants to survive in an increased bountiful manner. This supports cultivating an improved way of increased natural food production.

Millions of people struggle struggle for life's basic necessities. Sustainability and permaculture—both systems that consider the whole—are becoming more popular because of the necessity of going back to living harmoniously *with* Mother Earth.

When we live harmoniously with Mother Earth, what naturally happens is all components of a system are far more likely to be considered. When humanity can do this on a worldwide scale, all people will thrive.

To create as optimal a system as possible, it is best to create action steps that are most conducive to supporting all individual components in that system. Such action steps can include forming committees to understand the impact on all components within an eco-system, designing systems that will optimize and work in harmony with another system that could be impacted, and having respect and consideration for *all* components within the whole.

Understanding the full impact on all affected individual components of a system facilitates a wholistic approach in creating or altering any given system. This results in having a more complete picture of what types of impact can or will occur. In doing so, one can better harmonize and optimize the required action steps to take. This offers a wholistic approach, which naturally promotes harmony.

Many systems are in place that are already doing the wholistic approach, through grassroots movements and through some mainstream companies. There are many more companies not upholding improved, wholistic-approached standards. We can try to alert these companies and attempt to break down barriers in communication to help facilitate positive change. There is, on an energetic level, a breakdown of the old paradigm in which these companies do business, and their non-harmonious way of doing business are being exposed.

It is through this exposure that people are becoming more aware of the need to create a positive wholistic approach when running a business or large corporation. This exposure results in people feeling an increase in discord and uneasiness. It is no accident that now many current business practices are being questioned and examined. A new generation of workers continue to come forth to offer new and more wholistic ways of approaching how to run a business that is more in harmony with Mother Earth, as well as being in more harmony and respect to the company's employees and customers.

There is a need to have the old systems and inadequate paradigms be exposed. Through this, more people are becoming aware of what paradigms need to change, so that there can be an increase in proper alignment, resulting in increased harmony across our planet. This is why you see the movements like Occupy Wallstreet fighting against the 1%, why financial systems are breaking down, why there are more uprisings occurring, and why there is so much questioning of the existing systems. All this supports the entry into the new evolutionary leap into the new earth.

It is up to each person, as well as each business and corporation, to get into proper alignment, to live in tandem with what humanity is crying for, which is a new order, a new way of life. This new way of life represents the proper alignment and harmony with Mother Earth and with all of life. This new way of life yields the ability to optimize *living together* with other people and with humanity's host, Mother Earth. The new order of the planet and of humanity requires the harmony, respect, the gestalt, and in tandem-type living. Life on the planet will not survive otherwise.

Everything in existence is vibration and frequency. Humanity's vibration is currently low. This is due, for the most part, to the dominance of emotions such as anger, hate, fear, distrust, and other lower vibrational emotions. What humanity is being called to do now is to shift from this lower vibration into an increased dominance of higher vibrational emotions such as love, harmony, respect, and kindness. This shift of increased higher vibrations and associated higher vibrational emotions that are becoming more widespread throughout our planet, is one of the main components that will bring humanity into the much-needed new unity paradigm of our planet.

In order for this increase of vibration to occur, many old systems that are no longer working well, are breaking down.

They cannot stay in place in the midst of these higher vibrations. Indeed, we are witnessing many old paradigms breaking down. The new earth can best house only those living organisms that fit and match what is now becoming more and more the dominant vibration of love and harmony. The old cannot live in the new environment because it does not fit. The two vibrational types rub against each other because they are not of the same vibration anymore. Mother Earth's vibratory changes are such that it cannot comfortably house life that is not in harmony with her anymore. Mother Earth is coming to a place of less and less tolerance of her mistreatment. She is expelling out—a throwing up, if you will—the parts that cannot be digested. This is why there are increased occurrences of hurricanes, extreme bad weather, massive fires, earthquakes, and other disruptive weather patterns.

Be encouraged, however, to know there are effective actions you can take to make positive change. Some actions you can take are in section three of this book.

The Necessity of Change

It is through the various dimensions, or the different grades of *perceived* reality, that defines life's consciousness. For example, humans currently live in what we know as the third dimension. This 3D is a certain level, or grade, of conscious awareness that happens to be quite narrow and limited. It is in this narrow 3D bandwidth of perception that facilitates how humans live and carry on in their day-to-day lives. This results in creating a certain perception of what they see, and know, as reality. For humans, this narrow bandwidth of third dimensional living is valid. It seems real. It is, to some degree, truth. The key words here are "to some degree." It is actually not the full and complete reality.

The full and complete reality, which includes all dimensions, all grades and levels of consciousness, is in the realm of The Creator. There is a term called the consciousness vantage point, which describes the perspective by which one is conscious and aware. The consciousness vantage point for The Creator is complete and all inclusive. It includes all of the dimensions and all grades of consciousness. Most humans only have a limited consciousness vantage point due to the very nature of their being in the third dimensional level.

By design, humans came into existence to experience this particular 3D level of consciousness. In addition, by design, Mother Earth is here to house this particular life form's consciousness. Throughout the history of Mother Earth, there have been, and continues to be, planetary shifts. These shifts occur in particular cycles, and currently, as previously mentioned, Mother Earth is experiencing a 26,000-year cycle and shift. This is by design as well.

There is no accident—all is intentionally planned—that the Age of Aquarius is upon humanity now. And by design, systems such as the financial, economic, and government systems, are faltering. This is because the level of consciousness on the planet, and with humanity, is shifting and ascending. These systems that once could fit into, and be in alignment with, the energies and vibrations with the previous status quo cannot exist here now because the vibrations and energies have changed on Mother Earth. Life forms that are not in the same vibration find it uncomfortable and cannot exist in a container that is not meant to hold the old paradigm of life as we have known it.

We all have free will. It is certainly up to each of you to choose to come into alignment with the higher vibrations and energies. If you do, you will feel better because these higher energies are conducive to housing life in the higher vibrational state. Those who resist the higher vibrations or fight against them will find it more painful and difficult to live in this higher energetic environment. They will put up a fight to stay in the old paradigm. By its very nature, when this happens, there is a void, a nothingness to hold onto and the person finds it all the more difficult to live in a harmonious manner.

Today, the governments of many countries are in turmoil with the energies of conflict, so much so that there is little progress for good. The systems breaking down are such that the masses are impacted in a negative way. The word negative is used here to indicate the lower vibrations of it. These lower vibrations are keeping those energies locked and kept in existence, rather than having higher vibrations of love and healing thoughts. The higher vibrations would free up the lower vibrations of false beliefs, pretenses, negative emotions, and the old paradigm ways of thinking and being. What is best is to apply the higher vibrational emotions by many people to help dissipate and heal this, resulting in releasing these energies more easily.

The birthing process of this shift and evolutionary leap of humanity and of Mother Earth is not easy. It is painful. Those who are awake, such as lightworkers—the midwives of this ascension process—can and are assisting in this by living with higher vibrational energies. It is helpful to have even more people assisting now because there is so much pain, hate, war, and chaos.

In order for this negativity and disharmony to be healed, this negativity must come up and be right in our face, so we become aware of it. This has been, and continues to occur, and is one main reason for so much discord, pain, and upset. The next step in dealing with all this negativity is to fully feel the negative emotions in order to process them through. Once these are processed, they are much easier released. It is in the releasing of these energies that facilitate the healing. This healing is necessary for the individual, for groups and communities, for institutions and corporations, as well as on the global level.

In order to live comfortably and compatibly in an ascended consciousness and environment, it is necessary for people to be entrained with Mother Earth's predominant state of love, harmony, and respect because people are an integral part of Mother Earth.

The way in which people become entrained to the new earth's environment is by raising their vibration, and this occurs by living with love, compassion, respect, and a reverence for life. As this occurs on an individual and planetary level, the natural effect is that the lower vibrations of anger, hate, violence, and other negativity cannot survive; this lower vibrational energy can then be released and dispelled on a collective consciousness level.

When a person lives in lower vibrational emotions, it is difficult for them to survive and function well because living with those lower vibrations rubs against the fabric of the new earth's predominant ascended consciousness state of being. Those old, negative lower vibrations must continue to be pulled out and be released and neutralized. One way to do so is through people experiencing great pain, such as the various mass shooting tragedies that have occurred over the years. When tragedies such as these occur, the collective consciousness's lower vibrations have a chance to be pulled out and transmuted. The way to accomplish this is quite difficult and painful but is a necessary, and planned, action step for many people so as to continue with the ascension of Mother Earth and her people.

There is a natural order of things that must take place in the time and the manner in which they do, for this is a way to amend, fix, and rectify the millennia of years of humanity's ego fixation, separation perspective, intellectual and male dominance, competition, and disrespect toward life.

The movement of the change upon humanity is one of such critical impetus, that unless the necessary change of living in a higher vibration, higher consciousness and Oneness Living is taken upon by most people, humanity will become extinct. This birthing process of ascension takes time to complete, where the creation of increased higher consciousness is vital to go into the new state of affairs; the new status quo.

The settling into this new higher consciousness and vibration evolutionary leap will take time, and it will happen. With many of the awakened people such as lightworkers holding a high consciousness and high vibration, there is hope. Much work is still needed however. It is vital that the discipline to keep the momentum of light and love continues. This includes educating people to understand and to live from the perspective that we are all interconnected and to release their own personal negativity (we all have some). It also includes informing and educating businesses and corporations to operate with increased sustainability, cohesiveness, collaboration and consideration of all components within all of their systems, along with operating in a kinder and respectful manner toward all those involved.

The Deep Pain of Humanity

Every one of us puts forth a certain vibratory resonance and frequency influencing those around us and the planet. Like attracts like. You see, it is in the vibrational frequency being put forth that enables the surrounding areas to bend and flow, like a sea of fluidity. This allows for the expansion of life to continue. And life knows only one thing, expansion! Expansion is most effective when people flow and move with change, rather than resist it.

Imagine a rubber band that is easy to pull and bring back in. Rubber is malleable. However, if there is resistance, this rubber band does not move so easily. It can become stiff, perhaps stagnate and motionless. The same is true with humans. Their resistance to the evolutionary leap into higher consciousness and the Oneness perspective adds kinks to the whole. From this, a ripple effect is created, experienced as strife, unrest, and even more difficulties than can be imagined, which further contributes to more strife and unrest. This resistance is felt, usually on an unconscious level, by everyone because of our being energetically connected with all of life.

Let us take this analogy further. Imagine adding a ball to the rubber band and trying to catapult this ball by using a stiff rubber band. It is not as effective as a malleable rubber band. With the stiff rubber band of resistance, the ball gets stuck and is not able to move forward. Because it is stuck, it grows stagnant, and brings forth a stench that comes from being unable to freely move and not being able to expand. In a similar way, the planet is undergoing this stench, known as violence, war, greed, terrorism, and fear. This has created an increase in lower vibrational energies, making it harder to have the natural flow of life such as love, harmony, and respect. It is far more difficult to bring cohesiveness and proper balance to this stuck ball of humanity.

What can be done? Have more people living with increased love and kindness, compassion and caring, both for themselves and for others. Little by little, this optimal living will loosen up the stiff rubber band of lower vibrational energies. There are more and more people awakening to the benefits of living with a higher consciousness and the Oneness perspective. It is this awakening by more and more people that is softening the stiff rubber band. When there is a continual stream of this positive and high vibrational consciousness, the rubber band continues to soften and through this, movement and expansion more easily occurs. This brings forth the light of Divine good and the propensity for harmony. As the rubber band becomes malleable, the ball more easily catapults through the air in great joy and lightness, bringing more fluidity to humanity.

This is a stream of consciousness being cultivated now, through prayers, love, and compassion as well as an increased number of people becoming awake to the requirements of the new earth. As even more people become awake, the tips of the scales lean more toward peace and harmony. Cleansing out the pain and unrest is still required to alleviate negative emotions both individually and collectively. What is necessary to spiral up the ladder of ascension is the continual feeding of the higher vibrational emotions along with the awareness of Oneness, the interconnection of all life. When humanity accomplishes this—and it will—there will be a much-heralded peace that is so deeply craved by humanity.

In recognizing humanity's patterns of tyranny, abuse, lack of reverence for life, greed, control, hurt, and abuse, there is something important to understand. In all its accord, the masses have come to define these patterns as not being good. In terms of what we see as human suffering, this is difficult and painful to experience and to witness but it is imperative to realize that these circumstances have occurred to bring forth a cry from humanity to say, "No more! Enough! It is time to unite! It is time for positive change!" It is in the darkest hour that people bend and release. For when there is enough pain there is a softening in one's heart, for the heart no longer wants to suffer. It yearns for the innate longing of peace and of connection to its Divine self. This is where humanity lies now. There is so much pain and despair felt in the undercurrent of the river of life that lies in the furthest and deepest area of one's beingness. It is this area that is crying out for help. Both individually and on a collective basis, we no longer want to live with what does not *feel* good. We want to get into accordance with harmony, joy, and peace. We desire to be in alignment, unification and positive flow with The Creator and with our brothers and sisters on the planet. We want the stiff rubber band of resistance to soften so there is fluidity in life and increased ability to expand in a harmonious manner. With this, the life force of The Creator can easily flow unencumbered through all of life without strife, without bumping into stagnation or kinks so optimal living can occur including having the balance between the feminine and masculine restored to a healthy equilibrium.

There will come a time on our planet when you will see in history books the great pain, the great human revolution being broken through, the conquest of this leading to the great era of peace on our planet. But the times before are of great suffering. It takes this great suffering to birth the new. People are much more willing to take action steps for positive change and transformation when they are in pain. Like a caterpillar in the stage before becoming a butterfly, a complete breakdown of its essence occurs in order to *become* the butterfly. This is exactly what is happening with humanity.

From Out of the Ashes Comes Gifts and Rebirth

As we have just shared, humans are far more inclined to make a shift when experiencing great pain, tragedy or heartache. It is no coincidence that the world experienced the coronavirus pandemic. This is yet another wakeup call to humanity to take positive and effective action now! To create an improved way of life, we must all do our own personal healing; businesses and other organizations must start working in a sustainable, wholistic and cooperative manner, and all of us must also unite together to create positive global transformation. Why? So that we survive, not just a pandemic, but survive as a species for generations to come. Our very existence is at stake if we do not heed the call to take positive action now.

Yes, there was great pain and fear surrounding the coronavirus of 2020. Many lost their jobs, some lost their lives or loved ones. The global economy and personal finances were negatively impacted and social distancing caused feelings of isolation and angst.

And yet, once again, our species proved to be resilient. Many lessons and gifts were received from this crisis. Here are just a few:

- Creative ways to connect with others, such as singing to neighbors from balconies.

- A huge outpouring of volunteering and of monetary support for those in need.

- More prayer and meditation circles.

- Increased awareness of and gratitude for the blessings in life.

- Personal time for stillness and contemplation.

- Inner reflection of what really matters.

- Increased awareness that we are all in this together.

- Old wounds arising for us to release and heal.

- Mother Earth getting some rest by our slowing down from the daily busyness and frenetic energy we put forth.

- Positive environmental changes, such as drastically decreased air pollution in big cities and waters becoming clear in the canals of Italy.

- Businesses working with their customers on deferring payments.

Could it be that the coronavirus global crisis was the very impetus needed to wake us up? Is it possible that humanity's collective consciousness was crying for change so we could have harmony and respect, collaboration and understanding for all? Are you now a better person and do you now offer more compassion, kindness and respect as a result of the pandemic? Do you now feel more unity and interconnectedness with your family, your friends, your neighbors, your community—with all of humanity?

Clearing Out the Old
Supports Positive Change

We are being called to step up our commitment to change through the evolution of the next step of humanity. It is law that there are ever-changing evolutions, that organisms grow and expand. Energy cannot remain the same for long. It is vital to realize the profoundness of this statement! Growth and expansion must take place in the prescribed manner to ensure the expansion occurs in the way it is meant to, creating the needed energy change to support a more peaceful earth. Each person following their own path of higher consciousness can lead to positive energy changes, supporting the whole of humanity to move forward into the evolutionary leap.

How do you contribute to the necessary path of evolution? One main way is by clearing out old karma, patterns, habits, beliefs, and pain that no longer serves you. It is in the healing of these that lightens the load of the energy body of your physical body, which can increase your vibration and also open up your heart. Each of us expands and goes through positive change when the baggage of the pain's stagnate energies within the human body are lightened and released. This is, and always has been, a natural course of life.

This individual level of expansion through release and clearing out of that which no longer serves is another example of the micro versus macro level where the elements from all the individuals (micro level) conglomerate and pool together as a collective contributing to the whole (macro). When there are a large number of awakened beings contributing to the collective, humanity as a whole becomes lighter and of a higher vibration. This transformation is the endeavor of the day and is happening now on Mother Earth.

How do we ensure this path is taken by more people? You cannot account for others but you can account for yourself. It starts first with your being aware of the need to clear out and release the old paradigm and old ways of being that no longer supports or serves you, then to be committed to taking the actions to release this. Be aware that you may need to find support with a friend or a professional therapist to help you heal by clearing out the old patterns, habits, beliefs, or pain. We can choose to make a conscious positive change, and in doing so, we free ourselves to experience a more joyful life.

As more people are involved in their self-healing, others will follow suit. The reason for this can be explained with what is known as the Hundredth Monkey Effect. This is the theory stating that new behaviors will be taken up by others, once a *critical number* of people (or animals) behave in a certain way. This theory is based on the phenomenon that a primatologist discovered in Japan with Japanese snow monkeys. In 1952, scientists provided these monkeys with sweet potatoes covered with sand. They liked sweet potatoes but not the sand. One female monkey found a solution to eat them, by washing them. Other monkeys started to take on this behavior in a short amount of time. What is so startling about this is that it was discovered in 1958 that colonies of monkeys on other islands far away began washing their sweet potatoes too! A wonderful domino effect occurs; when more people realize the need to release the old ways that hinder them, others will start following suit.

In our current shift toward the new earth, more people are transforming by increasing their vibration and having higher consciousness, some through clearing out of their old patterns, beliefs, karma, and pain that no longer serve them. People are also realizing they are the creators of their own lives. The natural outcome of this is more connection with, and living from, the space of divine light and love. Living from the space of divine light and love simply means intentional living from the heart space and less from the head space (ego). It also includes being more often connected with The Creator. The ego is best used in life when led by the heart instead of the other way around. When living mainly from the ego, there is an inclination to perceive life as separate. When living predominantly from the heart center and from love, the ego will have less of a stronghold than it has now.

Humanity is being called upon to live life from the open heart, and one way is through clearing out the old to make way for lighter living and increased connection and higher vibration. This shift from the head to heart living will greatly shift all of humanity so that the orientation of life as a whole will be more peaceful. The new earth!

Renewal of Life

It is in the opening of the heart that allows for new experiences to come in, allows for new awareness to develop, and allows for new beingness to be created. Living from the heart brings people the space, the energy, and the vibration needed to create new brain neuropathways, which in turn leads to new beliefs and can create an environment that opens the brain frequencies to receive new knowledge. In this, there are physiological and emotional changes and this brings forth the necessary changes within the human psyche to experience life differently; we create a new reality for ourselves through this.

When you are willing to open your heart to the concept that we are all interconnected, you contribute to a positive willingness to believe in this concept and you also contribute to the collective consciousness. What will support humanity as a whole is to wake up to the realization that we are all one and in awareness of this truth, we gain more appreciation for ourselves and for *all* life.

There comes a time in each person's life to dismantle the old paradigm and to shift, change, move forward, and expand into a new way of being. A renewed way of life. This also happens on a collective basis. This mass movement is happening now and in this mass change comes destruction resulting in new life. For new life cannot happen without destruction. The reason for this is that in order for the universe to expand and change (new life), there needs to be a dismantling of that which no longer fits and no longer vibrates at the same frequency as it did in the old environment. Through the catalyst of change comes rebirth, bringing with it the seeds of new generations and new life. There can be no other way. It is the law of nature to break down and renew.

Think of a forest in the spring, which represents the renewal of life. Before this, there is winter; the colder temperatures are the catalyst to the leaves falling. It is the leaves falling that is analogous to the destruction and the dismantling of the existing paradigm (tree). When the leaves are no longer there, this allows for the new growth, the new leaves to come in the spring, for how can there be new leaves in the same place as the old leaves?

In a like manner, what is happening on earth now in the most unprecedented time of humanity and the planet, is that there is the change and dismantling of the old paradigm, the old vibrations and old ways of being. There is exposure of corruption and the old ways are crumbling, which makes way for the new. In this new comes a higher level of consciousness for both Mother Earth and for all of the life she houses, for higher consciousness is a natural forward progression of what happens when evolution occurs. Evolution is always in an upward motion and upward direction so we can appreciate the forward movement of change.

Those who are not in resonance with the planet's current conditions and new atmosphere have a difficult time adjusting and may fight against this. Their ego may be battling within itself, resulting in creating an inner war. It is this inner war that so many people worldwide are experiencing, and because this impacts humanity's collective consciousness, this is perpetuating the *outer* wars, that is, the wars currently happening on our planet.

While this collective experience of inner war is happening, there is at the same time an ever-increasing new status quo and paradigm being created, and that is love. It is in the difficulties of mismatched resonance between these two, that is creating the havoc on the earth, the people, animals, and plants. This is one reason for the extreme natural disasters that are happening and continue to happen. This is a reaction and phenomena to the two different energies bumping up against each other; like a cold front hitting warm air, the two conflicting energies cause a storm.

When those people of lower energy and vibration open their hearts and increase their positive vibration, change can begin for them and for the collective consciousness. It is in the opening of their hearts that neuropathways in the brain can begin to shift. When the heart is open, it is more in alignment with the new status quo/paradigm and new atmosphere of the planet, and of the many people of higher vibration and love causing a melting of discord and disharmony. Through this, calming and being more in alignment with the new higher vibrational ways occurs and this creates even more awakened souls on the planet.

How do you encourage and help others to become awake? Through your own healing work and through your own heart opening. It is by example and also by entrainment that those who are ready will follow suite. It is through this rebirthing of the planet's new higher-level consciousness that brings more people into the required alignment of this higher consciousness. Through this, there will be even more of an atmosphere of love. The dominant force on the planet will be love, so long as the masses continue to awake; when this happens, even more will awaken, leading to the tipping point toward a higher probability of worldwide peace.

How can one who is inclined to move toward awakening do so? What can you do to help? How can you open your heart and increase love in your life? Are you willing to learn new ways of thinking and being, such as understanding and living the loving qualities of The Creator? You, as well as those around you, benefit from this and you are also contributing to the collective consciousness. When you have daily practice of heart opening, you bring with you the increased resonance and vibration conducive to the new earth. In this way you create the frequency contributing to the collective frequency of love, and this acts as a type of magnet—the more people who become awake, the more of this power and magnetized energy comes into existence, which then creates more attraction, until finally there is a shift, a pop, a large mass, that is the predominant force by which the whole planet entrains upon.

Much happiness can grow from the perspective of living life with an open heart and the higher vibration of love. This is the new way of being and living on the forthcoming new earth.

Changes in the Greenhouse

The changes and shifts occurring on the planet are accelerating the light within each person. Many are being awakened. It is through this ascension process that allows for an easier transition of the light bodies of each person on the planet; and in this, they are better able to live with more respect for themselves, all living things, and for the earth.

As more people awaken, there is more love and caring for others and for *all* of life. Appreciation increases, even in the midst of the throws of negativity. As this love and appreciation continues to happen, the pivotal tips of the scale occur, as described earlier with the Hundredth Monkey Effect. There is no turning back.

There will be more peace on the planet due to the rising consciousness. What is this rising consciousness? It is the rising of vibration; the higher the vibration, the closer you get to the highest vibration of all, which is love. It is this arena of love that creates and facilitates living from the place of The Creator. For when living from love, there is no room for fear, hate, war, or destruction; only love's high vibration holds the reverence and the respect for of all life. It is within this love space that all people can better *see, feel,* and *know* the real truth of life, that all life is in unity with everything and everyone, that all life is important and to be respected and appreciated, and that all life is unfolding for the purpose of expression and expansion.

When living from fear and ego, there is more of a sense of being stuck in life, instead of flowing in alignment with life. Due to the very nature of fear and ego, it cannot perceive life as being interconnected. Fear and ego perpetuate a sense of separation. It is this sense of separation that creates difficulties, such as the deepened sense of individuality (instead of unity), the "it is all about me" mentality or the concern *only* about the company's bottom-line profits rather than considering the company's actions on *the whole* and all parties involved. The focus on the ego mentality, by its very nature, negates the perspective of wholeness and the interconnectivity of all life. It ignores *all* components that are interrelated.

Life cannot work this way harmoniously. The ego and fear-based living cannot exist any longer if humanity is to survive. As Mother Earth ascends with higher vibration, there is an increase with the planet's discord and an increase in violence. This is due to the ever-increasing mismatch of ego/fear and the higher vibration of Mother Earth. As Mother Earth's vibration increases, due to the ascension process, her environment changes. As her environment changes, it becomes even more difficult for Mother Earth to house lower energy frequency and vibration. It is like a greenhouse. Plants thrive when the greenhouse is at the right temperature and moisture, but when the greenhouse's conditions change, if the plants can feasibly and timely adapt to the greenhouse's new conditions, there will be a higher chance of surviving that new environment. The same is true with the planet now. Mother Earth's conditions are, and have been for some time, changing. People are adapting to it. Those living from lower vibrations, have an adaptation that is not congruent with the rising vibrations, and therefore are rubbing up against the new conditions. This is painful and is causing disturbances. It is causing a ripple effect to all. The sensitivity of Mother Earth to these ripple effects causes the natural disasters to be intensified, for Mother Earth's energy field picks up on the lower vibrations. The energy fields between humanity and Mother Earth overlap and interpenetrate, so naturally one impacts the other and vice versa.

Mother Earth is purging the lower vibrational energy, which continues to build momentum that continues to need expulsion from Mother Earth's energy field. In this way, Mother Earth is cleansing. This is analogous to a human who has taken on negative energy from someone else and needs to do an energy clearing to clear away the other person's negative vibration.

Those who are awake, who realize the changes on the planet and who come from love and peace, are providing the needed impetus to clear away the negative and lower vibrations. They are doing this by giving love, peace, harmony, and respect to life, which as you will recall, are the qualities of The Creator and are of the highest vibration. It is in this realm of Oneness Living that real peace resides. Those residents of Mother Earth radiating out Oneness Living are perpetuating the ripples of love to others, helping to displace the fear and ego. It is like a tidal wave of love, which is moving debris out of the way. A cleansing results. The same is now happening with Mother Earth.

Humanity is going in the direction of self-destruction, but as more awakened people and lightworkers help to displace this, there is hope that even more people will come forth with their calling. The call now is to continue to put forth high vibrations individually and also by gathering in pairs and in groups.

Love or Fear

There is much unrest on our planet and in this there are the seeds of potentiality, for the unrest creates the impetus for change. In this impetus for change, there is the creation for the behaviors and antics of society to bring forth the necessary changes to bring reform to the existing paradigm. The existing paradigm is no longer useful and cannot exist in the ever-increasing vibratory changes Mother Earth experiences. As was discussed, the greenhouse analogy explains that the conditions on the planet were once appropriate for the life that was housed by Mother Earth. Now that the conditions have changed, people must accommodate and acclimate to those changes. If not, those who are not acclimating have great difficulty in living, experience more resistance and tension, and also have more of the rubbing up against the new earth; they experience less flow and more chaos.

This is exactly what explains the ever-increasing hatred, war, terrorism, upset, and discourse experienced on earth now. This resistance and tension causes discord in the individual and also the individuals' sense of separation increases. Their fear increases as a natural consequence of the enhanced ego activity because ego operates from fear.

It is only through living in the higher vibrations of love and being in the heart space that the ego hold is lessened. What do we mean by ego hold? It is the orientation and perspective toward life that believes we are all separate from each other and that there isn't enough food, water, resources, and money. In other words, fear. A sense of separateness is perpetuated and this thwarts a person's ability from appreciating and *knowing* the truth that we are all one.

When a person is anxious, fearful, upset, or worried about not having enough food, water, or money, or when they are scared they might get mugged or they are concerned about the negative circumstances in their city or the world, these low vibrational emotions often build up tension and stress within that person. Most of the time the building up of tension and stress occurs slowly over a period of time and the person is often not even aware of the subtle changes of that increased stress and tension. Often living this way becomes the person's status quo, their normal way of showing up in life.

People do the best they can to try to maintain their status quo and whether they realize it or not, the stress and tension associated with this is also maintained; to do this, additional energy is required to continue holding their way of life along with their stress and tension. It becomes difficult to maintain this way of living, and therefore the person lets go and in doing so, much of the tension and stress energy are released. The nature of this released energy is conducive to discord, hatred, violence, disharmony, and also sustaining the perspective of separateness. Why? Because the tension and stress were born out of anxiety, fear, worry, and other low vibrational emotions. If it had not, the tension and stress would not have been created to begin with.

Let us take a look at a person who is with little or no tension and stress and usually has a minimal amount of lower vibrational emotions. Their way of living is generally more of a peaceful and happy one. This person is more relaxed and tends to go more with the flow of life. By being in an open heart space and love, these higher vibrational emotions contribute to the flexibility and relaxed state of living life. In doing so, this contributes to and makes it possible to more easily offer kindness, respect, and love to themselves and to others. The natural consequence is calm, assuredness of love, and relaxation as a predominant way of living. What naturally emanates out from higher vibrational people is a soft calming energy versus the sharp letting go of built-up tension. This built-up tension rubs up against, and is in sharp contrast to, the higher vibration of Mother Earth and to those who are awakened.

It is in the practice of meditation, love, an open heart, kindness, and respect toward all that sustains those who are living life from a place of love instead of fear. It is also in the love of yourself and the kindness bestowed upon yourself that maintains your relaxed state resulting in the ability to then put this forth to others. It is not selfish to start first with yourself because when you do you will treat others better. You see, it all starts with the individual person: YOU! You and those around you positively benefit. Can you see now why this information is vital to know? Would you be willing to make the necessary changes in your life to feel more relaxed and go with the flow of life?

Each of us are individual components and expressions of The Creator, just as the individual drops of the ocean make up the very ocean itself. When you start within yourself, this radiates out to others. Imagine an individual drop in the ocean living predominantly from the space of love, which is living from a higher vibrational state. Now imagine that the majority of the ocean's drops are living and being this way. This results in the quality of the ocean's atmosphere (in this case, humanity's consciousness' state) being healthier and more conducive to harmony and kindness rather than of the lower vibratory energies of hate, fear, and disrespect. When there are more drops in the ocean being and living in these higher vibrations, more love is propagated.

Imagine the drops have a color component to them and that the darker the color the lower the vibration. When more individual units/drops/people carry within them the negative or lower vibrational emotions, the ocean will be darker. Conversely, when more individual units/drops/people carry the higher vibrational emotions, the lighter and clearer the ocean (aka the container) will be.

This is an insightful analogy to understanding what you see today on our planet. Much of the discord you observe is the result of the many drops of negative lower vibrational emotions (fear). But when enough lightworkers and others who are awake, continue to put forth their light and higher vibrational individual drops (love), it causes a positive change in the environment, the container known as Mother Earth!

How does one maintain or get to a higher vibration? It is, in theory, simple: love one's self and you will love others. Love others and you love yourself. This, unfortunately, is not so easy or possible with many people on the planet now. Their upbringing, their set of circumstances, their ego-stronghold, their culture, their stubborn holding onto the old all contribute to less love and more violence within. And when this perpetuates, which it has for centuries, it creates a muddied-up environment/ocean/container, which is not so easy to see through. Fortunately, it takes less droplets of the higher vibrational emotions and energy to dilute and cleanse the muddied-up waters. This is why the awakened ones and the lightworker's positive work is so potent. Their higher vibrational states of being contributes much to cleaning up the debris in Mother Earth.

Now is the Time for Transformation

When we start with ourselves, we start with the world. For we are all in unity and connection. Our modality of being on this planet is such that we created a sense and an illusion of separation. This was set up this way to embark on creating a journey back home to The Creator, through understanding and living the Oneness and unity perspective. For it is the *experiencing* of life that expands our souls and through expansion we become heightened in our capacity to love.

It is up to you to choose the journey you call life, how you choose to approach life, and how you perceive a person or situation or how you see your life's experiences.

You are like malleable clay. Through your cultural upbringing and beliefs from childhood, you are formed as a piece of clay is formed into its unique shape. The sculpture's hands, as the clay is on the potter's wheel, goes up and down and in certain moves with the hands and sometimes with specific moves with the fingers and thumbs, the unique shape of the clay is made manifest into a ceramic bowl, vase or any other number of objects. So, too, do you create or manifest the unique shape of who you are with your perceptions, values, beliefs, thoughts, attitudes, words, and actions. Many of these came from your childhood and they are also created or changed throughout your lifetime. Each mold then further engrains the shape of you. The more often you think similar or same thoughts or verbalize these into words out loud, the deeper the physical grooves in your brain are created—the pottery of the mind so to speak. The clay is malleable to a point and then it takes on a final shape by being put into the firing kiln. But is it in the final shape? Not really. Yes, the fire's purpose is to put the finishing on it, but then this shape, now complete, gets handled, and in time subtle changes can occur, although these subtle changes do occur over some time and may be awhile before the changes are noticed. But they are there, such as a small scrape here or perhaps a crack or chip there.

You are indeed always creating. To optimize this, it is best to be *aware* of your thoughts and feelings, as well as the words you say out loud. This results in living more mindfully and helps to easier create your heart's desires.

There are circumstances that occur in your life that facilitates change and growth. And through this growth and expansion, we return home to The Creator. For in your innate beingness, you have a homing device to return to the arena of The Creator. You then begin anew with another life on planet earth, or you may decide not to; your soul is always evaluating and growing as it sees fit. Through this, your soul may decide to experience more on the earth plane.

The Creator extends Itself to experience a unique expression of Itself; and so, the cycle of life (as your 3D mind perceives it; in truth, life never ends) begins again, and does so with the birth of a new-born baby. The influences, beliefs, and values held by the parents are shared and imprinted upon their child, as the potter's hands imprint and shape the new fresh clay. As the child's uniqueness continues to be shaped, they become their own unique personality where their ego identifies itself with this personality. It is through this formation of personality that the child goes out to the world in which there lies many opportunities to create and to interact with others.

All the while the child's own thoughts, beliefs, values, and repeated spoken words are creating their own reality. This is because each of us are of the same vibrational essence and energy of *all of life*, in which whatever we think, feel, and act is vibrationally sent out like a radio wave to the ethers, also known as the imprintable medium or the field of infinite potentiality. This imprintable and malleable medium then, by the law of attraction, brings back to the child that which the child has been mainly thinking, feeling, saying, and acting. This is, of course, true for people of all ages. What we put out comes back to us like a boomerang.

You come to the planet as a newborn with a certain agenda on what lessons you would like to learn on this earth plane school. Each of us have a role to fill, within our families, our community, and, yes, also on the whole planet. And it is in playing this role in which we live out our life's purpose that all of us are here to learn what we came here to learn and it is always in perfection.

Nothing can stop you from experiencing what you came here to be and do. The beliefs, values, and perspectives you gained from childhood that were imprinted upon you, and carried forth into your adulthood, all support you in experiencing what you came here to experience. Even as you have thoughts of a certain perspective, and you experience what is *labeled* as difficult, it is still your intention to experience what you set out to do. This intention may or may not be on a conscious level. This is where mindful living comes in handy. It is best to live mindfully with intentions that you desire to see come to fruition. Many people live life unconsciously and therefore live life with unconscious intentions. They do not always realize the manifestations they are creating but the soul does have a way to steer the person back to the path they are meant to take.

For example, let us say there is a young man who is an alcoholic. He is here to experience what is labeled as difficulties that arise as a result of being an alcoholic. Once he finds he no longer wants to live this way, he is given opportunities, people, and circumstances that assist in changing the alcoholic behavior and he shifts to a different way of living. The whole experience is perfect and on purpose. The soul, through this, expands and grows into what he intended, not necessarily consciously, but intended nevertheless. The soul knows and guides him to what is needed to play out the experience of recovering from alcoholism.

Each soul on the planet is here to play out some experience or experiences to achieve the intention of growth and expansion into what the soul came here to learn. Just as the example about the young man's experience with alcoholism, and how his life took on the *intended* direction of a life free of alcoholism, each of us are guided to experience what we set out to do in this life's incarnation.

If you could see and know from the perspective of The Creator you would see the interaction, interplay, and synergy of all the souls (the whole) combining into one large collaboration of achieving the goal The Creator has for Itself: expansion and creation. For it is the purpose and intention of The Creator to do just this. It is through Its own expansion (through individual lives) that The Creator gets to know Itself. We are part of this intricate, vital whole. Without each of us playing our part in The Creator's intention/purpose of ever expansion and knowing Itself, the whole would not be complete. It takes *all* of us to complete the whole. If you were not needed, you would not be having your life here on the planet. You see, it takes each of us to complete the whole. It is best to do so when in harmony and alignment with The Creator, which expresses through each one of us. The ego fights this, thinking it is in charge when in fact it is not.

The current situation on the planet, which has also been true throughout most of humanity's history, is that most people live mainly from their ego instead of living in alignment with The Creator. Many people have their ego in charge, which slows down the ability to be in true alignment with their authentic selves and with The Creator. Ego is important because it assists in living in this 3D world of linear time and space. But for most people, ego has taken over their lives to the extent that they are not in alignment with The Creator and they are not living from their heart space. This causes havoc, as demonstrated by the state of affairs currently (and in past history) of the planet earth. This shows well how the ego has gotten out of hand, how ego bounces off of other egos, and how deep fear continues; difficulties continue to be perpetuated and created from the stronghold the ego has on them. This is evidenced by the war, famine, greed, self-righteousness, and the sense of separation that is so prevalent now, and has been for most of the history of mankind on this planet.

Living from the heart, and living with ego—by being influenced by the heart—is the optimal way to live. It is best to tame the ego through this heart-centered living and develop a healthy balance between both the heart and the ego. Each of us can consciously choose to transform ourselves to live more from the heart because we are malleable like clay. Each of us has the capacity to contribute to creating a more peaceful world through conscious mindful living, awareness of our thoughts, feelings, and words, along with using tools to support opening our hearts and living from higher vibrational energies of love, kindness, respect, gratitude and harmony.

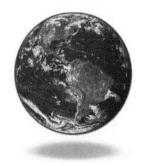

SECTION 2

Oneness Living

The Interconnection
of All Life

M any have an understanding there is separation among individuals. In some ways this is true. Each one of us has a unique set of traits, gifts, and personality that does distinguish us from others, and this uniqueness is necessary to the whole of life. It is like we are all an individual piece of a whole puzzle, contributing the necessary piece to make the puzzle whole and complete.

Yet, in truth, all of life is interconnected. How? Because at the most elemental level of all life, everything is energy. It is an all-pervasive field of interpenetrating energy that is also called the web, ether, matrix or the field of potentiality. This universal energy is the most basic source of all matter, animate and inanimate. It cannot be cut up because it is actually an energy field. What you observe, with your 3D senses, are pockets of concentrated, denser energy. These are comprised of a certain combination of atoms, which are, of course, also part of the energy field. Atoms emulate and show up as a particular item, such as a table, a mouse, a human, cement, a tree, a mountain, or the moon and stars.

There are many scientific studies proving there is this all-pervasive field of interconnection between all of life.

For example, in the book *The Field*, by Lynne McTaggart, several studies are sited. Here are two of them:

Edgar Mitchell, an astronaut, conducted a human consciousness experiment during the Apollo 14 mission in 1971. He randomly copied numbers; each being associated with Dr. Rhine's symbols that they agreed to work together with. Then Edgar concentrated on each of the numbers for the purpose of transmitting these, to see if Dr. Rhine's team down on earth would be able to pick these same numbers, to see if there was a match. It turns out this experiment was successful, with a 1 in 3,000 probability it was due to chance. The results of this is in line with the thousands of other similar experiments held by Dr. Rhine and his team. Being able to conduct this experiment from the moon to see if telepathy would work over a very long distance was an extraordinary opportunity.

By the way, some years after this experiment in 1971, Edgar Mitchell experienced an irregularity on his kidney. He chose to use a type of long-distance healing, an alternative to Western medicine. After six months of this healing modality, his kidney irregularity was completely gone.

In 1993, the research coordinator, Roger Nelson, Ph.D., for the Princeton Engineering Anomalies Research (PEAR) started using a random event generator (REG) machine for many of his scientific studies. The REG is a generator of sequences of random and unpredictable numbers that are then stored data in a computer. The purpose of these scientific studies was to test whether a person could influence this sensitive machine's randomness in generating numbers. If there was an influence on this REG, it would generate, statistically speaking, more NONrandom numbers.

Through a variety of experiments, he later realized he could use this machine to see if there is a statistically significant change in the REG's numbers with groups. If so, this would indicate there is group coherence. Group coherence is when there are many people who are together doing the same thing, such as a football game or a music concert, influencing the energy vibration of the group.

Dr. Nelson found that there was a definite NONrandomness that occurred during times of the height of a humor conference, a pagan ritual, and a conference's keynote speaker. These studies indicate that there indeed is a collective consciousness, as demonstrated by the statistically significant change registered in the REG machine during a group's like activities.

Gregg Braden, in his book *The Divine Matrix*, shares several scientific studies demonstrating the interconnectivity of life as well. One describes a 1993 study done by the Army. This study's purpose was to determine whether emotions affect the body's DNA, following a separation of the DNA from the body. The researchers collected a swab of a tissue and DNA, and measured the DNA in a different room from the tissue donor, to see if it responded to the emotions the donor was subjected to. What was found was there was a powerful electrical response by the DNA *at the very same time* the donor had elicited various emotions at different times!

This same experiment was done the same way, by the originator of this experiment, Dr. Cleve Backster. This would indicate there is some sort of connectivity between the DNA and the donor of that DNA.

Dr. Jeffrey Thompson, a colleague of Dr. Cleve Backster said it quite well: "There is no place where one's body actually ends and no place where it begins."

The energy that gives life to all life forms is known as universal life force energy. This is part of the all-pervasive energy field. Many cultures speak of this universal life force energy. In the Chinese tradition, it is known as chi. In the Indian tradition it is called prana and for the Japanese, it is called Ki.

The experience and feeling of the state of oneness and connectivity is a condition that people instinctually long for, strive for and very much enjoy. It is what people do on a conscious level when they seek community, for humans are social beings. Examples of this are when an individual seeks out a friend, a couple seeks another couple to eat dinner with, or a person goes to a community event, joining their community in song and dance. This longing to belong is what satisfies the innate need to be with, feel, and experience the union with The Creator.

When a man and a woman come together during love making, there is a combining of energies in which the chi (universal life force energy) of each person coalescence. There is a feeling of being connected with the other, where one does not feel a separation between them, but rather, they feel a union with each other and also with The Creator. The closeness and the total focus in the present moment of the experience with the other person in this love making brings a focus of interconnection between the two partners. This is why it is so pleasurable, because it creates for each person the feeling and sensation of being at one with The Creator, while being conscious. In a deep meditative state, whether through meditation, ritualistic dance practices or other forms of what may be called "altered states," are also means by which to experience the feeling of connection with The Creator. Many describe these states of oneness as being in bliss.

The tribes of India focus on the communal dances as a way to bring nirvana, experiencing bliss of connection with one another and with The Creator. They bring with them the keys of friendship, communion, elemental rituals to enhance and cultivate the synergistic experience of wholeness naturally. In the same way, Westerners will bring the connection through cultural traditions, such as weddings, funerals, and high school graduations.

When we realize we are all energy at the most elemental level, we begin to understand that indeed there is much more than meets the eye, for there is much that we cannot see, touch, hear, or feel but it is there nonetheless. Take gravity for example. You know it exists because you experience it every day. There are other phenomena demonstrating the interconnectivity of life that most people experience, including thinking of someone and then receiving a call from them. What explains that tense feeling you pick up on when you walk into a room just after two people have been arguing? When someone is gazing across the room at a person, and that person suddenly looks toward the person gazing at them? How do you explain the behavior of animals sensing an oncoming tsunami, the changes of fish behavior under certain ocean conditions, or birds flying in unison? Many people have had extrasensory perception (ESP) experiences, some of which were unexplainable. Other examples include the love felt between two lovers, and the sense a mother has when, 2,000 miles away, her daughter is in a car accident. The examples go on and on.

All emotions and states of being radiate out from us to our surrounding energy field and to the collective consciousness. So, whether you have love and kindness in your heart or have hate and jealousy, those emotions radiate out. People and animals pick up on these, some consciously and some unconsciously. We are all in this together, one in our connection. This is why we feel the pain, or the triumph, of another. We *feel* this due to the underlying "elixir" called the field, web, matrix, or all-pervasive field. It is that which interconnects and interpenetrates *all* of life.

Improve Life Through Oneness Living

The energy field, which we have seen, interpenetrates through all of life throughout the universe, and is what you may consider that which "holds" everything in the universe together.

As you have just learned, in the most elemental form, life exists as a flow of energy, an ebb and flow in what can be described as the sea of the field of potentiality. This sea of energy is so much more, as scientists have been discovering. There is the element of divine intelligence, a consciousness that orchestrates the ebb and flow of all life. It is the consciousness (some call it The Creator) that orchestrates how the energy field will take form. This form comes in many ways, including humans. Humans take on this consciousness, and in fact *are* this consciousness. Inherent in this consciousness is creativity, which exists via the field of potentiality, and is also known as the field of infinite possibilities.

The practical day-to-day applications of humans living in the 3D world is such that there is a perception of feeling and experiencing separation from all other life forms, such as other people, Mother Earth, animals, and plants. This human perception and sense of separateness provides a certain vantage point.

It is this certain separateness vantage point that most of humanity has developed into a vibratory overtaking. What this means is this separateness perspective is the dominant way of living for most people, and this has caused most of us to forget that we are all energetically interconnected with each other. Recall that the most elemental building block of all life is actually a field of energy. This is why everyone is connected with everything. Throughout thousands of years, humans have forgotten about Oneness Living and therefore do not live in a way that supports this perspective of life.

For so many, the need to cultivate oneness and community has disappeared. You can see this with large corporations that only have the stockholders' interest in mind, with no concern for the workers, nor for whatever impact it causes to associated components of the whole system related to the corporation. Scientific evidence has shown there is a lot of harmful exposure of radiofrequency electromagnetic fields to people and animals, with the new 5G technology, yet corporations are implementing using this anyway. We also witness the separateness perspective through the raping of Mother Earth, and many of its plants and animals; the lack of concern and respect for many people which pervades many cultures; and destruction through nuclear weapons, wars, tyranny, and treason.

To be sure, these examples of the separateness attitude and living would greatly diminish if the concept of Oneness

Living, that is, living with the knowing we are all inter-connected, are the dominant thoughts, beliefs, and actions of the majority or ideally *all* people on our planet. In doing so, there would be vibratory harmony with all people as well as the land and the plant and the animal kingdoms. All life would be in an improved proper balance and alignment. Discord, war, hate, and terrorism would be greatly reduced as a result. Can you now see why it is imperative that each of us transform our beliefs and way of living into the perspective of unity and oneness consciousness? Globally, we would facilitate a more peaceful and joyful world.

Imagine people throughout the whole world putting forth positive acts, deeds, thoughts and acts of kindness toward one another. Science has proved that what we put into the collective consciousness (via our thoughts and actions) effects change, so when the dominant thoughts and actions are positive, everyone around you will benefit. This supports causing even more people consistently living and offering their higher vibrational emotions and positive acts. If you and millions of people worldwide were living this way consistently, we would all—through our individual contrib-ution—effect positive change in a small yet important way. Collectively, in a large way!

Remember, all of our thoughts, feelings, and actions, whether they are of higher or of lower vibration, contribute to the collective consciousness.

The Influence of
Vibrational Energy

As described previously, the way for The Creator to know Itself is to constantly expand, and to have many expressions of Itself through this expansion. It is vital to understand that each unique expression, whether it is within nature, a human being, or within human constructs such as cities and government, is part of the whole. Being part of the whole means that what goes out (through action and thoughts), comes back to us (because we *are* part of the whole), and what is inside of us (our beliefs, our inner conflict, our vibrational energy) goes out to the collective consciousness.

One of the main ways we impact the whole is whatever we do to another person, animal or to our dear Mother Earth, we do to ourselves. When we remember all of our energy interpenetrates with all, we better understand that what we do and think affects others. For we realize our actions impact the whole. For instance, have you noticed when you are in a great mood and are friendly and kind with others, you tend to attract more people who are also this way? When a sad person walks into a room, they unconsciously put out their negative vibes, and other people tend to avoid being around that person because they do not want to pick up on this lower vibrational energy.

When large areas of the Amazon forest are cut down, the short-term effect is profit made for those involved with the deforestation. The immediate negative effect of the elimination of so many trees is also the elimination of the homes for all the animals, plants, birds, and insects that lived in the area. Consideration of the whole has not been taken into account. The long-term effects of deforestation are land erosion, which impacts the water drainage; and, like a domino effect, this negatively impacts the rivers and the people who live in the area. The inhabitants living here are also affected from these long-term effects. The people who were responsible for deforestation could well be the very people ending up being affected by their actions. Trees provide oxygen and with a large number of trees having been cut down, the consequence of this is less oxygen, therefore making a negative impact on a local level as well as on a global level.

When we consider the tendency of mankind to create war, we are able to assess the magnitude of its impact on the world and on an individual basis when we remember each of us contributes to the collective consciousness through our interconnectivity. Energy goes this way and also goes that way, meaning what is inside of us also influences the outside, that is, the collective consciousness.

Look within yourself to see how you create your own inner wars. Perhaps you battle within yourself regarding your belief that you are fat so you fight with yourself on what foods to eat, you are critical of your look, you create inner discord by constantly being stressed with your long to-do list, you may have money worries, you may be angry with loved ones, and so on. You fight with your car, you are anxious you do not have the perfect job or home, or you are upset about doing chores. You deny your own certain personality traits that you abhor. Because of your various inner wars, you may find ways to numb the pain of all your upsets, but these upsets do not disappear and they do not get resolved this way.

No wonder there is so much upset and violence on our planet! The majority of people worldwide experience internal strife to varying degrees, causing humanity to continue to experience discord and fighting. On the other side of the coin, there are many people putting forth positive energies that also contributes to the collective consciousness. Some global examples of this are the huge outpouring of love and compassion for the 9/11 victims and their families, the worldwide financial aid support for those affected by the number of natural disasters that have been occurring, and the millions of people who united together with social distancing to minimize the spread of the coronavirus pandemic.

Do you notice when you are around people you may tend to pick up on their mood? If you pay close attention, you will notice your mood may change to match theirs. You can choose to deflect any negative energies by being positive (although this may be easier in some cases than others), or as appropriate, de-escalate the person and/or situation of negative vibrations. Social workers, for example, generally hold a positive container for their clients, no matter what their client's mood is. When two people continue fighting, the intensity of the negative emotions increase due to their feeding off of each other's vibrational energy of anger. When you are at a party and it is lively and positive, you will tend to experience this positive space as well. These are all demonstrations of how our vibrational energies—due to our energetic interconnectivity—influence those around us, and also contribute to the collective consciousness.

Expansion of Life

What would it take to bring humanity around to a perpetual state of love and peace? What would humanity's state of consciousness need to be to experience the state of well-being with all your relationships at work and at home, understanding and respect across the globe, flowing with the harmony and the grace of The Creator?

It is possible to cultivate the new earth with these attributes. This would require most, or ideally all, people to emulate and live the qualities of The Creator. The qualities, as was previously shared, are kindness, respect, joy, love, harmony, gratitude and peace. Heaven can be made manifest on earth when you live your life by these qualities and also have Oneness Living.

How do you come to this state of love and peace? First, it takes knowing yourself and knowing your intrinsic divine nature—you are made in the image of The Creator. You experience your life in physical form, and at the same time, you are always connected with The Creator since you are divine nature. This is due to The Creator being the whole of everything, which of course includes you! As we have said, the very *nature* of The Creator is to create, and It does so through perpetual, infinite expansion of Itself, in individual form. *You are part of this!*

The different life forms, from single-celled amoebas, to plants and animals, to the highly complex life forms such as humans and dolphins, are simply varying degrees of energy. All of these life forms have one thing in common: they originate from one source, The Creator!

It is through the individualized expression of each life form that perpetuates expansion; through this, life knows life. There is a rhythm and flow of life that pervades everything. There is order in all aspects of life. Even in the midst of what seems to be chaos, there is order. There is order in the midst of all the life upsets, discord, and difficulties. When you can embrace and accept all the discord in your own personal life, you will better appreciate the natural expansion and the growth of your own life. This expansion and growth pushes forward your natural expression of what defines your purpose and expression in this particular life incarnation.

Through diligence and awareness of the growth you experience, you can then blossom into and live your authentic self! This growth is a microcosm of the macrocosm, in which you emulate the expansion of The Creator, only on a smaller scale. Expansion within expansion. Since there are billions of souls on our planet, each experiencing their own expansion, this adds to the collective consciousness' experience; this intrinsically and naturally expands The Creator's experience of Itself.

Through this expansion, we can experience the peace that we all want, both inner peace and world peace. Imagine with me what our world would be like when billions of people take active steps in their personal expansion. Personal expansion can look like healing your childhood wounds, thus making it easier to take on and live with the higher vibrational energies of love, kindness, joy, and respect. Personal expansion includes completely releasing all of your inner grievances, resulting in having substantially less frequent negative emotional vibrations of hate, jealousy, anger, anxiety, and other uncomfortable emotions. Personal expansion also includes Oneness Living; living with an open mind and heart and experiencing self-love and self-appreciation.

The result of many people doing their healing work will lead to more people experiencing inner peace. As always, when an individual person experiences any type of higher vibrational emotion, this adds to the collective consciousness, which results in a far greater likelihood of worldwide harmony, love, and peace, as well as expansion of humanity toward the new earth.

So, you see that when you work on yourself individually you are contributing to the creation of perpetual peace on earth.

Balancing the Spinning Plate

The time has indeed come to make changes on the planet. The ways of the old paradigm continue to shift, dismantle, and be destroyed. From out of the ashes comes the new age of humanity, known as the Age of Aquarius and the new ways of living continue to be formed. This formation is due to the required evolutionary shift that is simply part of the natural course of events: the human experience. In this shift there are ways to purge the ways of living that have not served humanity for many millennia. In our quest for control and domination, the human race continues to feed the annihilation of itself. It cannot go on as it has without the extinction of homo sapiens and of many other life forms on our planet, as well as further destruction of our dear Mother Earth. Therefore, in order to make shifts out of this destructive paradigm, we must slowly dismantle the old ways of approaching life. We do this by offering optimal and new ways of being and by purging and releasing old energies. The release of the old pain and suffering can take many decades, but slowly the cleansing will be done and over the next fifty years or so, more light will emerge as the dark is cast aside and lovingly transformed into the ethers.

We can best approach our own lives with sanctity and honor our own way of cleaning out our debris of pain, hurt, and suffering. We must focus on ourselves and on this healing so we may further accentuate the planetary healing. As more people do, the momentum of planetary shift will increase and there is a real possibility of peace once again.

Yes, there was peace at one time on this Earth, about 200,000 years ago. Humanity can once again experience peace, given the right circumstances, the most important being that we remember—and live our lives by the premise—that we are all interconnected. It is imperative that many more people come to understand and experience this Oneness Living, for this will nurture creating the new earth so many are yearning for. This is the very reason why the message of oneness and love is currently so popular. As more people do their healing work, they free themselves from being encumbered with negative emotions, thus increasing their vibrational energies and experiencing a more joyful life.

There is an impetus to make change. There is an innate knowing within Mother Earth and within each person that the time has now come to make this change. It is simply law: the natural unfoldment of humanity's evolution. You can say it is like a child, who has within its beingness the ability to grow, get bigger in size and age, and turn into a young adult and then age more. The same is true with humanity as a whole. Humanity grows now into the next stage of its "life span" and so the cycle of life continues.

How can you help cultivate this natural innate expression of humanity's evolution? You can first start with expressing your own innate talents (if you are not already doing so). To do this, you must come to know yourself and become once again acquainted with your own natural inclinations and talents. Many of us have squelched parts of ourselves to the point of no longer being aware of them. Rediscovering yourself so you become reacquainted with all aspects of who you are is necessary to live more in alignment with your true nature, allowing you to live more authentically, that is, living closely to your true individual nature. Then this allows you to express your unique and necessary contribution to the whole. The whole world would flow more harmoniously when all of us live authentically. Certainly, there is much work to do before this ideal state of being is achieved. There are many healing modalities and personal development workshops continuing to come forth that help people achieve this state. Bit by bit more people are awakening to their true authentic nature. When critical mass is achieved— as explained by the phenomenon of the Hundredth Monkey Effect—there will be a worldwide shift and what a celebration on earth this will be!

We start with ourselves and this radiates out to others, for the vibratory nature of the universe is such that who we are contributes to the collective consciousness. The vibration, when higher, elevates the collective state of consciousness. In this symbiotic relationship between the earth and humanity, a state of interaction that cultivates the new earth is reached. It is this higher level of vibration that sustains harmony and peace.

Think of it like the juggling act of spinning plates on a pole. Once a certain level of speed and balance is achieved and sustained, the plate continues to spin in the way it is intended. If this state is not sustained then the plate starts to wobble, and the potential exists for it to fall. It is vital we continue to build velocity to achieve the momentum and height required to bring in the new earth. When enough people reach a state of awakening, the proper vibrational height will be achieved and the whole earth could balance and spin properly, in a manner that perpetuates and cultivates harmony and peace worldwide.

It starts with you! Follow your heart's longing; follow your internal GPS. It will never lead you astray. If you follow your own path and honor your own unique ways of being and live authentically, with love at the helm, there can be peace on earth, bliss and joy can prevail and in this there can be the highest level of evolution achieved.

Discover in this book's next section, the ways in which you can contribute to answering humanity's cry for change by starting your own personal journey of change and positive transformation. This can include: unloading that which does not serve you, increasing your vibration, living more consistently in your heart space to cultivate love, listening to your inner guidance, and recognizing the magnificent, divine nature of who you really are! Together we can, and will, answer the call to create and live in the new earth, which promises the joy and peace so many of us are seeking.

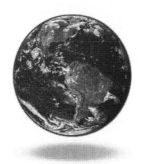

SECTION 3

Individual Opportunities for Positive Change

Maximizing the Benefits of These Exercises

There are many opportunities for you to experience the positive change and also the healing you desire. By using the following exercises offered here, plus the many workshops, self-help books, alternative healing methods, support from friends and/or professional counseling, and other modalities readily available, you will experience an improved way of living, heal old wounds, and increase your overall sense of well-being.

As you choose the exercises you would like to experience from the following pages, you will support your success in achieving your desired results from the exercises by first setting an intention for receiving the benefit from them. Making an intention is effective because it is a declaration stating what you want and expect. Intentions, like any thoughts and feelings you have, transmit a signal out to The Creator of what your desire is (because everything is vibration and energy), thus increasing the probability that your desire will manifest.

Another useful concept to optimize and increase effectiveness of these exercises for change and healing is to make a commitment to yourself to sincerely use these exercises several times a week or even daily.

Awareness of who you are, of others around you, of what is going on in your environment, and being aware of the present moment is key in all aspects of life. You are encouraged to also be aware of how you react and how you feel when using these exercises, as well as how you are benefiting from them. There may be some exercises that push your buttons, others that cause you to feel you are outside of your comfort zone, others that may bring a deep sense of relief, joy, or other positive emotions, and still others that empower you. Whichever way you react to and benefit from using these exercises, remember to be kind, gentle, and compassionate with yourself. And, embrace the change!

Keep in mind that, although there is great benefit to each of the exercises here, you may or may not also need professional support, such as from a coach, counselor or therapist. Different people need different levels of healing. Having awareness of where you are on the spectrum of life will support your knowing what additional healing modalities, if any, may be right for you. Are you in need of just a little support in increasing your sense of well-being and making positive life changes? Then these exercises may be all you need. Does your state of being require working through and healing deep childhood or family trauma/wounds? Then seeking the additional support of a professional therapist may also serve you and these exercises may very well augment your professional support. You may also seek additional support through talking with trusted friends and family. Be willing to explore and to trust yourself in knowing what you can do to maximize your desired change and healing.

Remember that as you continue to work on increasing your sense of well-being and healing, not only are you making a positive difference for yourself but you are also making a positive difference to those around you and to the whole planet, through our interconnectivity.

Have hope and excitement for yourself and for our planet as you step onto this journey of positive change and self-healing. Lighten your heart with the knowing that all is well prepared for you, that you are so supported in this journey that increases self-love, higher vibration, joy, and inner peace.

Raising Your Vibration

Raising your vibration from where you currently are will support you in your overall sense of well-being, help you relax more and facilitate having increased love, respect, harmony, joy, and peace toward yourself and others. Increased vibration will also help you flow more easily with life, rather than resisting it. Would this not be preferable over living predominantly from anger, jealousy, anxiety, guilt, and other lower vibrational emotions?

Certainly no one lives 100% of the time in the state of high vibration. Life's continual ups and downs provide an array of emotions and experiences. However, you can strive to live your life *predominantly* from this state of being. It takes time and practice to raise your vibration where this becomes your normal, predominant way of living. It is possible to achieve this with intention, commitment, awareness as well as determination and practice.

EXERCISE

Here are two exercises to raise your vibration:

Love Essence

You are invited to practice a morning meditation focusing on your heart space and having a remembrance of a "love" experience. Love experiences do not mean sexual, but rather, of a warmth and bliss of love, such as what you would feel with a loved one, like a mother or dear friend, or even a pet. For a few minutes or longer, have a sense of appreciation and love as you remember a love experience. Breathe this into your whole being. Now use your imagination that you are pleasantly saturated in this love essence. For example, perhaps you see yourself immersed in sparkles of love and light, or you feel a warm calm energy throughout your whole body. Next, set an intention to carry this feeling with you during the day.

Similar to this love experience meditation, you can bring forth your own love essence from within and then intentionally send this out. This not only raises your vibration but assists those close to you and contributes to the collective consciousness' state of being. How do you tap into your love essence? One way is that you can imagine a beautiful nature scene or remember the smell of something pleasing or act as if you are with someone you love and trust. Closing your eyes, invoke one of these suggestions and bring it into your heart. Feel it and be with it for a few minutes or longer, bathing in the sensation of this.

You will prolong the benefit of these (and other) exercises by setting an intention to carry the feeling with you as much as possible during the day.

EXERCISE

Present Living

Bring yourself the gift of present living, also known as the practice of mindfulness. This means be aware of, and live in, the present moment, the now moment, as often as you can. When you are truly focused in the present moment, you are not living in the past or the future, resulting in reduced worry about the future, and less regret about the past, resulting in you experiencing higher vibrations, increased calm, and mental clarity. You may want to read Eckhart Tolle's book *The Power of Now*, for a more detailed understanding of putting this important practice into your daily living.

Being mindful can include taking the time to enjoy where you are and to not rush yourself. Be willing to have more awareness of where you are at the moment by stopping and looking at a pleasant photograph of your loved one, smelling flowers on your walk, breathing in the aroma of a meal cooking, walking outside and appreciating the beauty in nature, and mindfully brushing your teeth or washing your hands. As you do any of these activities, do so with mindfulness, being fully present with the act of this present living.

Living in mindfulness also brings with it a better ability to surrender and accept what is, rather than resisting it. This offers inner peace and this in turn cultivates

higher vibration. Recognizing that which
cannot be changed, that which is in your control to
change, as well as viewing life's circumstances with
nonjudgment, will help bring you increased relaxation
and calmness, which cultivates higher vibration.

Sensing the Universal Life Force Energy

Each person is a reflection, a microcosm, a hologram image of the world. We each hold all elements of the world. This is true because we are all energetically connected through the universal energy field, the matrix of life.

We begin to understand this when we realize we are all from the same source, The Creator. Our lives are sustained and we remain alive through what was mentioned previously, the universal life force energy, also known as chi, ki, or prana. This universal life force energy is part of the universal energy field itself.

You experience chi energy in different ways, such as when you walk into a room and feel the high and positive vibration between two people in love with each other. Maybe you experienced holding someone's hand and felt a subtle tingling sensation. In a Reiki or a Healing Touch session, most clients feel calming energy. And many have experienced this energy through martial arts, chi gong or tai chi. All of these examples demonstrate the all-pervasive presence of the universal life force energy.

By you experiencing the chi energy within your own body, you will be able to better embody the concept of interconnection and unity. You will also be in more presence and awareness with yourself and those around you, which also supports you appreciating that we are all one.

It is easier to increase your awareness and be more present with yourself when you are in quiet meditation. Quiet meditation allows you to better feel the sensation of the chi energy in your body because you minimize any outside distractions and inner mind chatter.

Chi energy flows throughout your inner and outer body. It is contained in what we perceive to be boundaries of our skin. It ebbs and flows, interpenetrating with the outside environment, or what is perceived as outside; in reality there are no boundaries, just different levels of energy frequencies.

EXERCISE

The following two exercises will help you experience the sensation of chi energy:

The Physical Body's Chi

Sitting in your favorite chair, on the floor, or wherever you are most comfortable, relax and get into a quiet space within yourself by becoming totally present and focus on your breathing for a minute or so.

Next, set an intention to feel the chi life force coming through you and just simply be aware of the quiet space and of your body. Be an observer of yourself. The chi energy is subtle. It is possible for you to feel it, most easily at first, in your arms and hands. It may feel like a soft vibration or a humming or tingling sensation on your own skin or there may be indirect sensations. You may simply sense the quiet calm. Some people have described this sensation as a lightness, transparency, clearness, or a combination of these.

With practice, you will feel more of this chi energy. For example, you may feel it in your chest cavity or other areas of your body. Be open and patient as you develop an increased skill in feeling this wonderful sensation.

Even though you see with your eyes the boundary between your skin and the air, energetically speaking, there really is no separation. Seeing is not the only way to experience life. It does not always reflect reality because seeing is only a limited sense. For example, when you look at a loved one, can you see love? No, however, you can feel the love. When you gaze lovingly into your loved one's eyes, you can feel the love. The same is with your pets. Yes, you can see a separation from your body and your pet's but when you are in the total moment of play with your pet, or you are stroking your pet, you can feel a connection and you feel love. Many experiences cannot be seen, and you cannot see with your eyes the continuity of the universal energy field, yet you do experience this through other means, as just described.

EXERCISE

Sensing the Continuity of You

Be an observer of yourself by witnessing your awareness of the breath as follows: Imagine chi to be a flow of subtle current by focusing on your breath. Breathe in, and imagine the chi flow is moving up, then breathe out, imagining the flow moving down. Do this for several minutes. Now become aware of your heartbeat and at the same time be aware of the quiet and of any sensation of chi flowing through you.

Next, see if you can feel the end of your skin and the beginning of the environment that is right up against your skin. Can you feel it? No, you cannot, because there is no separation between the two. What you will likely experience though is a floating feeling. If you do not already feel this, be patient. You will sense this with practice.

With our busy day-to-day lives, you usually do not feel the chi energy. You are not aware of the boundary-less essence that exists between all things. However, when in the quiet of meditation, and also setting the intention to feel the chi energy during the day, you increase the ability to feel this. Consider making meditation and also chi awareness a daily practice in your life. Try this while you are waiting in line to buy your groceries. Set a time each morning for your meditation practice. Take a three-minute break during your work day to pause and then intend to feel the chi energy pulsing throughout your body. It is a wonderful way to come into more presence and awareness of yourself, which helps you relax and be more connected.

Your Life Purpose
and Inner Guidance

It is far better when making decisions and choices to do so when living consciously and being mindful. Through the decision-making process or with everyday living, you can better assess options or what is right for you when you are attuned to your feelings and emotions, and deciding from the heart instead of the head/mind. In this manner you are more following your true inner guidance system (also known as your gut feeling, intuition, or inner GPS) that has been put into place for you, by you, to mark your path, lighting the way so you can easier fulfill your life's purpose. When you follow your true inner guidance system, you will live more authentically, resulting in being able to apply your important piece of the puzzle to the whole of humanity. There are no accidents. You are here for a specific reason. You have come to play a vital role in the whole of humanity here on earth.

When you follow your inner GPS, you will find you *feel* better and the things you desire to implement comes easier to you. Why? Because the path is open when you follow your heart's desire and follow your inner GPS, versus when you go by your head and mind, which easily creates an obstruction.

It is through the heart and inner guidance that you can better implement the path that has already been formulated and laid out prior to birth.

There are lessons and gifts along the way toward fulfilling your life's path, and this is intentional, for they contribute to the fulfillment of your life purpose. In knowing what your heart longs for, and honoring its beaconing, you can better assess the legitimacy of the action steps required to bring forth the fulfillment of your life's purpose.

Let us consider an example to demonstrate this concept of fulfilling your life's purpose and how that is easier when following your inner guidance system. Let us say Joe comes into this life as a carpenter and wants to build homes. As a child he has always had inclinations toward working with the earth and with wood. He finds he mettles with wood, and has a natural talent with creating pieces of art through the wood he collects as a child. As a young adult, he finds he wants to create a living making wood cabinets. He has success with this way of working. He has followed his path and his natural inclination of working with wood.

Next, there is a man named Steve who has the same inclination to work with wood but his parents shy him away from it due to their belief that it is not proper for a son of a business man to go into the trades so he is forced into college to study a variety of topics, only to find himself severely disinterested. It gives him no chance to work with his hands and nature. He finds other ways to fulfill his innate push, by working in a bar making drinks and finds himself drunk night after night, because there feels to be something missing in his life. He cannot quite get his head around why his life feels empty, so he finds relief with drinking and getting drunk with friends.

There is an internal guidance system established within each one of us and when nurtured and honored, will allow us to open the gates to many opportunities and avenues in which to fulfill our natural inclinations and life purpose. You can say, we are wired to do certain things and if we do, we are more easily able to flow with our life's purpose. Deepening into trusting our inner GPS and knowing our true selves allows for more of The Creator to flow through us unencumbered!

The natural enfoldment of The Creator is to express and expand. This occurs through each one of us expressing our unique skills and talents and through fulfilling our life purpose. Imagine the whole world given the opportunity to do just this! The ebb and flow of life as a whole would be more fluid, harmonious, and collaborative. How to establish this worldwide flow of harmony and collaboration is the purpose of humanity's next step up in evolution, which is happening now!

Just as the individual is an expression of a unique aspect of The Creator, the whole of humanity is also an expression of The Creator, a whole organism so to speak. It is the macro level versus the micro level. Humanity experiencing its life purpose of leaping now into the next level of evolution is analogous to the individual person experiencing their own next step in their own life, leading to (hopefully) fulfillment of their life's purpose.

EXERCISE

There are several ways you can nurture hearing your inner guidance.

Nurturing Your Inner Guidance System

Pay attention to your feelings and emotions. These are the indicators of your inner guidance system. When you feel happy or positive, this indicates you are doing what is best for you; you are in alignment with your true self. Likewise, when you have a bad feeling about something or someone or are just feeling a negative emotion, this shows you are moving away from what you want and away from who you truly are. You may well want to avoid the bad feelings.

When you make a decision, ask yourself if this decision makes you feel happy or excited, or do you feel uncomfortable or uncertain? Honest exploration of your feelings gives you insight on whether the decision you made is the right one or not.

Another way to better hear your inner guidance is through meditation. Meditation as a daily practice quiets your mind, so you hear less mind chatter. In doing so, you will increase your ability to better hear your inner guidance and increase your awareness of your feelings and emotions, not only while meditating but also during the day.

Periodically during your day at work or at home, pause for a few minutes and become aware of how you are feeling. Do you feel happy? Stressed? Anxious? Is there an inner voice trying to get noticed? Perhaps your job is not satisfying, and when you pause and reflect how you *really* feel, you realize you are unhappy; your gut feeling tells you once again that you would prefer to switch careers.

These suggestions to improve hearing your inner guidance will take practice. You will find as you do that you will become proficient with this and improve your life immensely. Remember, it is listening to your GPS that supports your ability to live life more fully and joyfully.

Call Forth Love Through
Your Heart Space

When you have love in your heart, you feel better and you have higher vibrational energy. Those around you also benefit. Why? Because as scientists from HeartMath Institute have discovered, the heart's electromagnetic field is the strongest rhythmic field the human body creates, thus offering the heart's ability to extend out its energy field several feet in all directions. Since you are interconnected with all, your love energy field overlaps with others.

You no doubt have experienced feeling the heart's energy field in different ways, such as your interactions with loved ones, giving love to your pet, or feeling good energy from a group activity focusing on positive energy showering love vibrations from the many participants in that group.

EXERCISE

Here is an exercise to go into your heart space and create an increased feeling of love. This exercise is similar to the one on how to raise your vibration, however this one invites you to bring the feeling of love while you are not meditating, although as an option you can do that as well.

Opening Your Heart Space

Start by focusing on something or someone that makes you feel good and brings you joy. This could be your child or loved one, a pet, or a special place or activity, such as taking a walk in the forest or on the beach. You can think of a happy childhood memory, perhaps of a caring teacher or neighbor who spoke kindly to you. Create your own happy thought if you cannot think of any, just make sure it feels real.

Now, continue focusing on this happy feeling and act as if it is already happening. Perhaps you will even jump up and down with joy or excitement or you will stand up with gratitude. The mind does not know the difference between the real experience or just thinking of it; either way will bring you into this heart space. Once you are feeling this, you are causing a higher vibrational field within yourself. As you do so, a current or stream of consciousness is created, emanating forth from your whole being, with the heart being central. Be in this flow of positive heart and love energy for as long as you like and keep it with you during the day.

EXERCISE

Try out this exercise to both experience more of the love essence for yourself and also to share this with others.

Radiating Out Like the Sun

Once again bring yourself into the state of open heart, either through meditation or in an awakened state, and imagine the warm, soothing rays of the sun radiating out from your heart space. While doing this, imagine your vibration increasing. As you bask in these soft rays of sunlight, you are quite likely to sense the calm and peaceful feeling of this higher frequency called love embracing your whole body. Be with this for a few minutes or longer. Now imagine radiating this out to the room you are in, to the building you are occupying, to the community, the state, the country you are in, and to the whole planet.

Feel the love radiating out and be aware of the state you are in. Stay here as long as you like.

Slowly bring your awareness back into the room. Bring back the love essence to your heart and set an intention of your heart's desire, or make a prayer to keep the flow of this love with you during the day.

As was mentioned, being that the electromagnetic field of the heart radiates out several feet, you impact and touch many around you regardless of whether it is a positive or negative vibration. Therefore, it is beneficial for as many of us as possible on the planet to live from the heart space of love. This is one major way we can positively influence a change on our planet and to contribute toward a new earth of Oneness Living.

When you use this, or other activities that promote increasing love, your heart energy center (chakra) is open and pouring forth love energy. This love energy is the most elemental component, and of the highest vibrations, of The Creator. You literally carry forth the true essence of what The Creator is, love. In this state of pouring forth love, you will feel bliss, calm, and peace.

This type of activity can also be used by a group of people gathered together who have the intention to create the heart space energy and resulting love for the benefit of, say, victims of a natural disaster or for a family's loss of a loved one. There is a strong synergy of each person's love energy coalescing and radiating out together, making for an even larger impact on the people they are focusing this energy toward. It is through this commingling of the many hearts' energies that results in a higher vibration. It is as if you are turning on a light switch in which the group cohesiveness creates and generates even more power. A sequence of events is set off, causing momentum of the intention set forth.

World peace is possible when all people are predominantly in the state of the higher vibration of love. It is imperative that individuals step up now to create love in their hearts and live from this heart space. Those who can relate to feeling love from the exercise described above, or other ways, can uphold this for themselves and also for those who are not able to.

There are many who are hurting, who have never experienced love or have at one time, and now cannot feel it and have closed their hearts. Hurtful experiences can cover up the pure love essence. It is important to uncover this pure love essence through peeling off the hurt experiences that have tarnished and covered it. Self-kindness, self-respect, and self-support will help loosen up old wounds. Also, recognizing the good we each have within ourselves is imperative to keep this self-kindness, self-respect, and self-support going.

EXERCISE

You most likely have heard of the benefits of using positive affirmations or comforting phrases repeatedly. Why do they work? Because over time, your brain creates new neuropaths resulting in new positive beliefs. Plus, saying positive words in that moment supports you in calming down and intercepts negative thinking. It helps to redirect yourself into more uplifting and higher vibrational thoughts.

Here are a few, and you can also create your own. Remember when creating your own to keep them in the positive stance.

Self-nurturing Affirmations and Phrases

Close your eyes for a few moments and as sincerely as possible say to yourself any of the following phrases, offering comfort in the same way as you would toward a close friend:

I know you are doing the best you can.

You are a wonderful person.

You are doing ok.

You deserve a good day.

I am successful at my job.

I really am a thoughtful person.

I am kinder to myself.

I am willing to love myself.

I am now treating myself with respect.

If these or other phrases are not believable yet, continue using them. You may even want to add the words: I am willing to ... For example: I am willing to love myself. Your brain hears whatever words you say and by stating: I am willing to ... will support you in embracing this as new truth and beliefs about yourself.

Thoughts like these start a new thinking, and this in turn supports changing how you feel about yourself. Changes and releasing of old wounds are happening much faster these days, so the benefits of saying positive affirmations and phrases is quicker than in past years. With intention, consistency, awareness, and commitment to create greater self-love you will experience positive changes.

Perhaps you may feel the need to receive assistance in healing your wounds or upsets. As previously mentioned, there are many healing modalities through counselors, coaches, and psychotherapists. Personal growth workshops, self-help books, spiritual retreats, and also working with a trusted friend are options as well. Go with your gut feeling on what is best for you to clear out the old pain so you may heal.

EXERCISE

Here is an exercise for you to cultivate inner peace in a playful way. This will help you get started with having more self-love and inner peace as well as open your heart space more.

Playful Heart Space for Creating Inner Peace

Find a place where you feel safe and that brings you comfort. Be open and willing to talk to your heart and your inner being with love. Then use your imagination to playfully visualize you are pouring forth grace upon yourself. For example, you could pretend there is a pitcher of red hearts representing love being poured all over you. Allow yourself to be playful and make believe with this visualization of grace upon you.

Now breathe in this love. Soak it in. Allow yourself to

open your heart and feel the love essence inside of you. If you do not immediately feel the love, then just pretend and allow yourself to act as if it is happening.

Then be quiet for a few moments and listen. Hear any words that may come forth. Be patient, like when talking to a child offering understanding, kindness, and love. Now see how you feel.

Now imagine putting this love feeling into a special jar with a lid (either imaginary or real). Intend now to have access to this love feeling and that you can reconnect to this same feeling by taking the lid off or to peek inside to experience the same love sensation you created. Be playful while doing it. Pretend to hear laughter, or better yet, laugh out loud by the sheer joy of knowing you can access self-love and self-accepting feelings from this jar (or from anywhere), knowing you can always have it with you. Take a deep breath and be willing to believe you deserve this, for indeed you do!

Increase Self-Esteem and Self-Love

I It is not egotistical to think you are wonderful and that you offer great talents and gifts. Who you are matters and there is a reason why you are here! You, along with everyone else, are offering your important piece of the puzzle called humanity. It is absolutely important and actually even necessary, to feel good about yourself and to have high self-esteem and self-love. There are many attributes about you that you and others can appreciate and acknowledge.

What *is* egotistical is believing you are *better* than others or that others are beneath you. Many of us were brought to believe it is not ok to think well of ourselves. However, know, for your sake and humanity's sake, that *everyone is of equal importance.* When you feel better about yourself, not only do you feel better, but you also see the good in others. Remember, what you see in others is a reflection of what is inside of you. Do you see now how important it is to realize your greatness, increase your self-esteem, and self-love?

EXERCISE

The following exercise is a safe and gentle way for you to build up your self-esteem and self-love. It is recommended to do this daily, and even twice daily, to create a habit and to become accustomed to realizing the greatness of who you are. It only takes a minute to start, then after a while, you will find that a few more minutes every day will be beneficial.

Mirror Exercise

Daily, starting out with a few seconds (or longer if you wish), look in the mirror directly into your eyes, then acknowledge yourself for who you are, what skills you have, a positive outcome you experienced, or anything else that acknowledges the wonderful person you really are. Whether you believe this now or not does not matter. Doing this exercise is powerful and is safe to do.

Next, if you are willing, look into your eyes again, go into your heart space and think of a joyful thought. Now, send love to yourself from this heart space. Offer yourself this love along with compassion. Be with this feeling for a minute to start with. Increase the time of looking into your eyes by adding a few more seconds each day. Continue this practice over many days and weeks until you become accustomed to looking at yourself with the heart and eyes of compassion and love, and with support and acceptance. This will help loosen negative feelings you may have for yourself and allow loving feelings to enter. This is a slow, safe, and gentle way to become acclimated to yourself. This creates a conducive environment to feel safe to be with yourself and gently start loving yourself.

EXERCISE

This exercise will help you remember and embrace the positive attributes about yourself. This supports feeling better about yourself.

Contemplate Your Positive Attributes

Write down a list of experiences you recall having that indicate your positive behaviors and personality traits, and also helpful positive actions you have taken and compliments you have received. Perhaps a kind teacher who gave you praise, a neighbor who thanked you for helping her, your parents encouraging you, your friends commenting on how thoughtful you are.

Next, write down personality traits or attributes that you like about yourself. If you have a difficult time coming up with anything, think about your natural talents, what comes easily for you and/or what you enjoy doing. Do not be shy with creating this list; each of us have several talents.

Now, allow yourself to think well of yourself for having what is on these two lists of positive behaviors, personality traits, actions, and compliments. Contemplate them lightly and acknowledge yourself for them. It is best to do this exercise several times, even as a daily practice.

You are encouraged to now empower yourself with the belief that you *are* valuable and you deserve to think highly of yourself. It really is ok for you to do this!

Self-Exploration
and Authentic Living

One of the most effective ways to enjoy life in an optimal manner is to live authentically, for it is in authentic living that you bring forth the best of yourself. You live authentically by knowing yourself well, and by seeing who you really are and being ok with that. To thine own self be true: to honor and respect yourself in all regards. For when you have self-approval, others then also will approve of you and will interact with you in a more authentic way. Like attracts like, so when you are authentic you bring more people to you who are also authentic.

What does it mean to live an authentic life and be true to who you are? It means to bring forth those unique qualities that are the makeup of who you are. For example, have you known someone who feels happy and alive when they are expressing themselves with their gift? An artist who paints, a school teacher who teaches, a mentor supporting a child. You can feel their love and enthusiasm in the actions they promote. In contrast, when you see someone who is sad or neutral, one who just does their work for a paycheck, you can feel their unhappiness. Walk around in a public place and witness the expressions of people's faces. How many are joyful and have a sparkle in their eyes? Likely you may see more people who are unhappy than happy.

There are many people who feel like something is missing in their lives. This is often due to not living authentically. They may not be living their life's purpose or are not in alignment with their true selves. They are here existing in the manner that has brought a dis-alignment, a mismatch of their gifts and the tasks they are performing. Finding the spark in their heart, honoring and living their soul's mission would bring much joy.

If you are a person who is not living authentically, how can you address this? How can you be encouraged to follow your true and authentic self? It is in the discovery and the knowing of yourself and the willingness to explore yourself, that brings forth the awareness of your being, gifts, and talents. Through this exploration, you can then have a clear picture in your mind of what you can accomplish and what will bring you joy and excitement.

There are many people entrenched in the negative, so discovering who they are can be difficult. These people are to be commended for their fortitude for living, existing in the best way they can. They are doing their best. Everyone does. How can these people move forward? What can they do to change? Part of the answer lies in the ways we treat them, putting forth our love and healing thoughts. Offering some guidance and caring. Showing by action that they matter. Offering respect and support. Bringing to them that which brings forth their heart's desires. Show by modeling the advantage of knowing firsthand what it feels like to be in authentic living. Offer compassion, tools and teaching, which can lead the way for them. It is best for us to not only offer ourselves to ourselves but to also express our true selves for the benefit of others. Others will thrive more when we put ourselves forth in an authentic manner, that is, be true to ourselves.

Stepping into our authenticity means stepping into our grandness. To be big. To stand tall in who we are.

EXERCISE

Exploring Yourself

Take a piece of paper or go to your computer, and be willing to be honest with yourself. Create a list of your gifts, skills, and talents. If by chance, you cannot think of any, reflect on the positive compliments people give you. For example, "I love how you dress," "You are always so good with people," "You have a gift of writing," or "You have a magnificent garden." You can also think of any activities that come naturally to you, that are effortless for you to do.

Now, ask yourself sincerely: Do you consistently use your gifts, skills, and talents? If not, what has stopped you from doing so? What are you willing to do to start using them? In what other ways can you cultivate living more authentically?

Once you have the answers to these questions, for any gifts, skills, and talents that you would like to use or to use more of, write down the action items you are willing to take to do just this. Then determine a date by which you will have these action items complete. For example, perhaps you have a special talent in working with animals and would enjoy doing this through volunteer work. Set a date to meet the volunteer coordinator at a couple of animal shelters, to explore where you would like to volunteer. This will provide you the opportunity to live your authenticity by offering your talent of working with animals.

Living authentically and true to yourself also means to recognize, *and be willing*, to do the inner work to resolve any upsets or pain you may experience. There are many who are in a state of despair and they may not know which way to turn. For example, a person can experience difficulties with relationships with one's self that outpictures and manifests as difficulties with relationships *outside* of themselves. What outpicture means is: that which is *within* ourselves gets projected *outside* of ourselves. It is like a movie projector, projecting onto a screen that which is inside, such as a person's characteristic or personality trait. Say that Michelle is very confident, and she admires a close friend who is confident. Michelle's confidence is being projected outward, seen in her friend's confidence. You can only see in others that which is within your own self. Most of the time this is done unconsciously. Being aware of those people you most admire and also those you dislike will help you discover what is within you!

Those personality traits that are within you that you do not like, are ashamed of and/or are afraid to have someone find out about, are what is known as your shadow personality traits. Everyone has several shadow personality traits. This is because each one of us carries *all* personality traits within ourselves, some being more dominant than others. By now, you probably can guess why each of us has within ourselves all personality traits: because we are all one!

It is important to offer to ourselves and to each of our shadow personality traits compassion, to discover the gift that each shadow personality offers us and to integrate each trait into our awareness and beingness. In doing so, you become a more whole person, get to know yourself better and you can live more authentically. An excellent book to read for a deeper understanding of your shadow sides and how to positively work with them is *The Dark Side of the Light Chasers*, by Debbie Ford.

As mentioned, it is important to discover and know yourself. Recognizing what you outpicture is one way to do this. In knowing yourself, you can better appreciate how you act, react, and interconnect with others. Therefore, it is beneficial for you to establish a habit of continually getting acquainted with all aspects of yourself, including your shadow personality traits.

Here is an example of a woman named Jane who is a career woman with many ambitions, one of them being to make it to the top in a corporation as president. She finds herself struggling with her peers, because they find her too abrasive. Her attitude toward others is one of dismay and separateness, she is not a team player and she feels it is all about her and what she can glean from others without regard to their feelings. This brings a difficult situation to Jane in making it to a high management position, where in fact people tend to stay away from her. When we look at Jane, we see she struggles and battles within, not honoring or respecting herself. She acts and lives from a place of habit and rote without regard to her emotions.

Jane's unhappiness arises from the difficulties she had from her interactions with her siblings, always being out favored by her parents, and she felt she must compete with her siblings to get attention from her parents. This discord between her siblings and herself, the fighting for attention is what has caused her to act out in her job, with competing for attention by having the disharmony with her peers and within herself. Although she is good at her work, she finds it difficult to move through the required relationships.

If Jane were to examine the inner battle within herself, she would understand her sense of competitiveness and realize her need to have validation. Creating this sense of validation from within her, instead of from outside sources, she would find she can consistently receive this for it is an unfailing source from within. She would experience more peace and calm, which would naturally emanate from her and be reflected in the interactions with her office peers. To the extent that she is willing to examine the root cause of her behavior, honor it and respect it, is the extent she has of understanding and knowing herself better, which increases the healing of this inner pain and struggle. This in turn allows for a better appreciation and knowing for how to act with herself and with others. Coming to embrace this part of herself brings a realization that can bring the understanding that all behavior on the outside is simply a reflection of the inner dynamics from the inside. We can better recognize and be aware of our own nuances and realize this shows up in our relationships, our jobs, careers, and all other areas of our lives.

Recognizing the inner root cause of your nuances, patterns, and behaviors is true accountability and responsibility. It offers an improved and better way of living, better than from living with knee-jerk reactions, drama, unconscious living, and relationship difficulties.

Being accountable and living in awareness of yourself brings you the insights and understanding of your inner most beingness so that you can re-evaluate your behaviors and therefore make changes as needed. Be willing to look outside of you to the events and circumstances of all areas of your life, as well as what you are outpicturing. This will give you a deeper understanding of yourself. You become more peaceful inside and your outside world also becomes more peaceful. Why? Because that which is within you is what you see outside of you!

EXERCISE

Here is an invitation to you to explore even more about who you are. Keep in mind that everything you discover is absolutely okay! Do not judge anything you discover. You are, always have been, and always will be, a magnificent person whether you think you are or not! The real truth of who you are is always the divine spark of life, made in the image of The Creator.

Deeper Inner Exploration

Without judgment and with an open, compassionate, and honest heart, take a look around you and answer these questions: What do you see? Who are the people you associate with? What kind of job do you have and how is your relationship with coworkers and supervisors? What feelings do you have during the course of your everyday living when it comes to interacting and reacting to others? Do you have feelings of calm or angst within? What is your dominant state of being? Are you willing to explore the deep crevices of your being, so you can better understand all aspects of yourself, so that you can make peace with those parts of yourself that are in disharmony with you?

With eyes that are willing to lovingly and gently see deeply into your soul, continue to explore, to contemplate, to assess. You will be most pleased if you realize that all parts of yourself are of the divine and that The Creator always holds you in a positive light.

Next, go into your heart space and invoke the love you have, then give this love to all parts of you, even those parts you do not like. Through this find peace. Find calm. Find acceptance. If you feel you need support from a friend or a counselor, certainly make the time to get that. You are never alone in this.

At any time during the process of answering these questions, if you find yourself uncomfortable with continuing, then simply stop. It is totally fine to put this exercise aside and continue later. Do this exercise only when you feel ready.

Your Life Purpose
and Authentic Living

There is a river of life that explains the cause of each person's experience. Although unseen, this river of life, the undercurrent, the ever-present Creator is always pulling gently for you to go in a certain direction, to allow the goal of fulfilling your life's purpose. It is as if the higher consciousness is in charge—and it is—since you are a part of the all that is, The Creator. Recall that The Creator experiences Its expansion through individual life, such as you.

Imagine there are rocks in a river. Water runs into and then goes around these. It is the same with human consciousness, you. You experience your life's occurrences as the water in the river, running into, and then going around, experiences, challenges, and opportunities (rocks) making your way down the river. You are carried by the ever-present undercurrent (The Creator) while you are experiencing the rocks of your life.

When you go down the river in a relaxed manner, you can then move around the rocks of life's experiences, challenges, and opportunities easier than if you were resisting them. Imagine being in a boat and riding on this river, going along with the current but trying to avoid the rocks. You can do this, yes, but it requires more paddling and therefore more energy. Letting go of the oars can yield a smoother ride if you trust your boat will gently glide over those underwater rocks.

There are times in life when you do need to take hold of the oars once again. This could mean that you need to set intentions and take action received from your inner guidance system, to then use this guidance to steer clear of any obstacles. If there are rocks that stick up above the river's stream, it is best to steer clear of them. You do this by taking the boat's oars and work in collaboration with your internal GPS and with The Creator to know what to do to steer clear of them.

The same is true in life. It is better when you can steer clear of obstacles (rocks above the water) that do not serve you. It is important that you are aware of any obstacles that may exist in your life. You can use the oar of trust and your GPS to steer you back to the right direction, which is your designated path of life, your life's journey. In this way you can begin again with your travels on the river of life.

You can align with your own path and life purpose, and be ever mindful of what your path and life purpose is. You can establish a routine of dedication to your path in which you glide through your life with trust and faith, listening to your inner guidance system and also following your heart. Being persistent, committed, and mindful will keep you on the path you are meant to follow.

There are many ways in which you can perform your life's purpose. Recognize that whatever choices and actions you make to perform your life's purpose are fine. It is as the ocean refuses no river. You are always loved, cared for, and accepted by The Creator for whatever choices and actions you take to perform your life's purpose. Believing and trusting that all is well yields this to be.

Standing in truth of yourself and your conviction will build a stronger conduit, a portal, with which to pull yourself further along in your river of life all the while knowing that what is pulling you along is your connection and faith to The Creator.

You have life experiences that are meant to propel you further along toward fulfilling your life purpose. Often, you have no way of foreseeing the many events in your life; however, they are well-orchestrated by The Creator to facilitate your life's lessons from your experiences. This also supports deepening your wisdom.

Each day you become a new you through the cumulative experiences you gain through your life. What is most profound to understand is that once you come upon your own congruence, you can flow on the river of life far more freely and peacefully. Letting go of the boat's oars allows you to flow gently down this river of life. Be like an open door, allowing what wants to come to you, come. The keys to keeping the door open are daily prayer, faith, trust, focus, mindfulness, and relaxing. You will benefit even more when you exercise your mind to be diligent in its discipline to stay on track with these keys.

When you live authentically, you live more congruently to your own self and you are also making a positive difference to humanity by raising your vibration. As your vibration increases, the collective consciousness is positively influenced, which in turn starts to facilitate a more peaceful world. As you probably recognize by now, when you help yourself, you are also helping humanity.

EXERCISE

The following exercise will support you in exploring your life purpose.

Contemplate Your Life Purpose

Sitting comfortably in a chair or on the floor, allow yourself to contemplate the path and purpose of your life with honesty, self-compassion, and nonjudgment. Become aware of any diversions you may have encountered during your lifetime, or currently, that may have taken you off of your true intended life's path. Recognize also that you can once again go into the direction needed to fulfilling your purpose in life. Awareness of yourself and your path allows you to steer toward where you are meant to be so you can fulfill that which you came here to fulfill.

Perhaps you have not discovered your life purpose. If you are now willing, create a strategy to find it! You can search the internet, go to the library, find a workshop that facilitates discovering your purpose, or seek out a friend or counselor to help you explore.

You can also gain insight to what your life's purpose is \
by asking yourself:

- What compliments do people give me?
- What activities do I find enjoyable?
- Which gifts and skills do I have that come easy for me?
- What makes my heart sing?

If you know your life purpose and find yourself not living it, consider creating action steps that will bring you to living it. You can honestly answer questions such as:

- What obstacles, if any, has stopped you from experiencing your life purpose?
- What resources do you have to get you back on track?
- What action steps are you willing to take to get you there?
- What is a first baby step for you to start taking?
- What support system, such as a good friend or coach, can help you?

Next, write down specific dates by which you will have completed the action steps you choose to take. Find someone you trust with whom you can receive support in, and be accountable to, with accomplishing these action steps. As always, be patient, understanding and nonjudgmental as you do this exercise, and feel free to pause and start again later if you feel you need to.

_____

What is Working
and What is Not

When you are in the throes of a busy life, how often do you stop and assess your life by asking yourself such questions as: Am I happy? What upsets me? Am I in the right job? Am I living the life I am meant to live? What is my heart calling me to do?

All too often, people get accustomed to their own life's status quo that they may not realize they could be happier and have a more authentic life. Change in a person's life often happens so gradually that they may not even notice the subtle shift that has occurred in their life. They may find themselves feeling unsettled, unhappy or frustrated.

To assess your life and your state of being, you can do a treasure hunt. It is called a treasure hunt because you will begin to get to know yourself better, and this is a treasure in itself! Through knowing yourself better, and then choosing to take the necessary steps to move forward and create the life you dream of, you will indeed excavate the true you. You will tear down the walls that have kept you from living your authentic life. You may find the need to hire a life coach or counselor, or have a trusted friend to hold you accountable.

Here is an example of a treasure hunt. Let us say you are in a job that feels like a burden to go to every day. Start by asking yourself why you are still there. What elements of the job, the company and/or work peers are not working for you? Drilling down to as many specifics on what is not bringing you joy will assist you in bringing new light and awareness on what you are doing with your time and your life. The next step in this treasure hunt is to explore what career and work you would prefer to experience and that would bring you genuine happiness. Here, you can ask yourself:

- What activities and natural talents do I have that makes me feel fulfilled?
- What excites me?
- What have I always wanted to do but never have?
- What am I comfortable with doing?

Answering these types of questions will bring awareness to your mind and through this, you can then begin the next process, which is determining what you will need to do to get from your current situation to where you would rather be.

Brainstorm, think outside the box and use your imagination to determine what changes you need to make in your life. Allow yourself playtime in your mind. Through this you can begin to explore what action steps to take. It truly is an excavation of discovering hidden treasures as you are going through the process of this suggested self-exploration. The journey *itself* will bring many gems and diamonds to you representing expansion, growth, increased self-awareness, and self-knowing. And it is in this increased self-awareness and self-knowing that gives you the ability to see what is in front of you, so that you can then decide if you are willing to make the necessary changes in your life. If you decide to make those changes, you will create a life of authenticity and this leads to more events, people, and opportunities coming to you with increased ease and less effort on your part. This will increase your experiences of sheer joy, inner peace, fulfillment, and calm.

EXERCISE

Similarly, to the previous chapter's exploration of living authentically and living one's life purpose, let us now evaluate what is working and feeling right in your life and what is not.

Treasure Hunt

If you are willing, take an *honest* look at what is working for you and what is not working for you in your life right now, then through this self-exploration, you will find great treasures that can bring light to such questions as mentioned above.

Grab a notebook and pen now, or get your computer and sit down with an open heart and begin to explore your inner treasures. Be sure to remember to do this with self-compassion, nonjudgment, and sincerity. Have fun with this!

Refer to the questions above that support exploring yourself and also the above treasure hunt example for ideas to get started. Use your imagination and dream big. Something to be aware of is the inner critic most of us have that often pops up and says to you false statements such as: Who are you to have what you want or be who you really want to be? or You cannot do that. As these thoughts come up be aware of them, and simply acknowledge them. Then tell these thoughts: I do not need to listen to you! I know I can have my dreams come true! I choose to listen to my heart, and my heart tells me this new career brings me joy and excitement! I choose to live authentically now!

Certainly, making change into creating, and then living, your dream life will take time depending on what the changes are. But with every journey, each person needs to begin by taking the first step. The journey starts with that first step, and you can choose to do just this. It is possible to make the change in your life if you believe in yourself fully enough. In this, you will be able to create the stepping stones that will bring into fruition the desired life, career, relationship or any other area of your life you desire to make change in.

Imagine a world in which everyone takes action to live authentically. What would this world look like? How would people treat themselves and others? What is the outcome of a company in which the owner decided to bring her company to the higher level of social consciousness, the ripple effect of that company on its employees, customers, and affected aspects involved with the company's products or services? Imagine having millions of companies worldwide operating from this perspective. What would the world economy be like? Would the resource usage of the companies be sustainable or wasteful?

If the whole world lived in authenticity, this would create more pieces of the whole puzzle showing up. And in this, the intrinsic nature of the whole becomes stronger. For when all pieces are put in place, the whole becomes more stable, increased optimization occurs and the synergistic effect of all pieces showing up add to the collective consciousness' higher evolution. As a result, this leads to a more solid, stable, and balanced world; just as the whole puzzle becomes more stable and stronger, the whole Mother Earth becomes more stable and stronger.

Choose then, to excavate your inner strength by assessing where you are now and where you would rather be. Then take the steps and do the research and solicit the help of friends and family to help you move into your dream life. Together we can create a better way that will be in line with the new earth's higher consciousness and vibration.

Prayer, Faith and Belief

By praying from a place of love instead of fear, there is a higher vibration and you become uplifted. It also uplifts the vibration of the collective consciousness as you know by now.

It is best to pray from the stance of believing and being faithful that what you are praying on, or for, is already done rather than being fearful your prayer may not be answered. It is believing and having faith that are the key ingredients for the successful fulfillment of any desire. This is nurtured and fortified by praying from love rather than fear.

Prayer is a creative process. The act of putting forth one's desires through prayer places it onto the creative material of what is known as the ether, matrix or the field of potentiality of the universe. It is as if there is clay to mold your desires. Through this clay, it makes it possible to fulfill the desire or see the change you are praying for. It is through the intention behind the prayer that makes it more likely that that which is desired will come forth. To be in the place of faith and belief, along with intention, increases getting one's self into alignment with the source of all, The Creator. To use the analogy of a turnkey to demonstrate this alignment, imagine there is a lock that you want to open and you are turning the key. The key needs to be turned in such a way as to get it to click to be in proper alignment so that the key is aligned with the inner structure, the inner workings, of the lock. It is then that the lock is opened. The same is true with prayer; once you are in proper alignment with The Creator through intention, belief, and faith, what you are praying for can better come into manifestation through the flow of universal creation.

Another way to promote living in alignment with The Creator, as we have seen, is to open your heart, and through this, the vibration of love is accessed to a greater capacity. This, coupled with having belief and faith, gives you better ability to co-create with The Creator. Why? Because you are in an *increased connection* with The Creator. Remember, this becomes all the more powerful when you set a sincere intention and when you pray from the space of love instead of fear.

How do you increase faith and belief? How can you come into a deeper belief in The Creator, in life's process, in yourself, and in the co-creative process? You can start by going into your heart space to create a greater sense of love. Setting an intention to do so makes this process all the more powerful and effective.

EXERCISE

Pray with an Open Heart

The suggestion for this exercise is to pray in any manner you are accustomed to and that feels right to you. Remind yourself of the benefit of praying from love rather than angst, worry or any other type of fear. Opening your heart space will allow for more of your love to come forth, which naturally raises your vibration. Tapping into your belief and faith in any way that works for you is also encouraged.

Your Bandwidth

E ach of us have the ability to tap into our inner wisdom for guidance and insight on how to live our lives. As we have seen, this is also known as intuition, gut feeling or accessing the infinite wisdom of The Creator. Rather than being able to access *all* information, we have access to limited information for we are privy to only a certain amount of knowledge. This information that is specific to you and what you are to know for your life's journey is called your individual bandwidth.

You can easily access the information within your bandwidth by being connected with The Creator. This is done through different ways, such as daily meditation practice, following your feelings or gut instinct, opening your heart, and also by increasing and then maintaining your vibration to higher levels. By accessing your bandwidth's knowledge, you are riding the wave of an ocean, so to speak. Imagine an ocean with its many waves and you are riding on top like a surfer. You are being pulled by the very nature of the wave's momentum. The same is true when you live your life by "riding the bandwidth" (the wave). You are naturally pulled forward into the life you have come here to live, by using the bandwidth's information to support your decisions and actions, as well as gaining insight to your life. This propels you into a forward momentum, creating the unique flourishing and unfolding of you.

Contrast this to when you may not have tapped into your bandwidth's knowledge. You may have experienced a time in your life when your intuition was loud and clear, yet you decided to not listen to that inner guidance. You likely ended up feeling resistance, regret or upset around that time, as a result of not listening to your inner guidance. Likewise, perhaps there was a time in your life that you wanted to gain clarity about an important life decision that you were confused about. Being able to tap into the wisdom of your bandwidth could have provided the clarity you were seeking.

EXERCISE

Meditation is an effective way to develop increased access to your bandwidth's information. The following are some basic tips on how to meditate.

The Gift of Meditation

Daily meditation enhances the ability to have easier access to your specific bandwidth's information. Fifteen minutes of meditation in the morning, ideally also fifteen minutes midday, and in the latter part of the day as well, is recommended. When it is not possible to meditate three times a day, at the minimum, doing this once a day is good. For a wonderful way to become centered and alert during the day, take even five minutes to meditate. If you are new to meditation, start out with even just five minutes and then build up to a few more minutes over time.

There are many types of meditations including sitting quietly and in silence while focusing on your breath or heartbeat, walking in nature with great mindfulness and awareness of your environment (present living), listening to a guided meditation, stretching, and dancing. Any activity that supports you being totally in the present moment and focused on something is considered meditation. Find one or several types that you are comfortable with and that brings you deep into connection and centeredness. The important component of meditating is simply the act of meditation itself, for this allows you to experience the presence of The Creator, the reality that is underneath our busy mind chatter. With continued meditation as a daily practice, you will notice that over time your mind chatter will decrease. Have fun with your daily meditation practice by using different types of meditations.

What are the advantages of living daily with this entrainment to ourselves through daily meditation?

- You will become clearer in your mind as to what actions to take, resulting in experiencing an easier climb of life's natural unfoldment.

- You can easier access your soul's wisdom and guidance (within your bandwidth) in this state of being.

- You can better follow your assigned task in this incarnation, always allowing for a natural, organic progression of your gifts, offerings, and skills to the world.

- You have more authenticity when living in tandem with the wisdom within your bandwidth; therefore, you are happier.

- You create more relaxation and calm during the day.

- You have less mind chatter during the day, even when not meditating.

- You can easier deal with life's challenges and difficulties.

One of the ways to create more momentum and forward movement in your life into the direction you are meant to go is through the discovery and through accessing your life's bandwidth (inner wisdom). It is through this you establish your necessary foundation that holds you up and keeps you strong, enabling you to carry forth your unique and vital role to the whole world. Remember each one of us is an important and necessary piece of the whole puzzle called humanity. Your piece is equally as important as anyone else's. The whole puzzle (humanity), becomes even stronger, and there is an increase in stability and cohesiveness that is created when *many* also offer their authenticity. And as we have seen, this has positive and far-spread benefits worldwide. The dynamics of so many people offering their unique selves would be powerful and would encourage harmonious living and peace as a result of its optimal synergistic impact on the whole.

Now is the time to come more into your own alignment and to strive to love your own life as best as you can, living in tandem with your bandwidth. For in doing so, you are offering your vital piece of the puzzle to the whole.

Connecting to The Creator

All of us are already connected to The Creator. It is a matter of degree in how much we are living and feeling this connection as well as being aware of this. When we are awake, aware, and live more intentionally, we are more attuned to the whole unity of life, resulting in an increased connection with The Creator. This raises our capacity to more fully tap into the light of The Creator. The light is the very essence of The Creator. It is goodness, the absence of darkness and the shining love radiance of The Creator.

Tapping into The Creator's light is like an electrical light switch—the flowing electricity is always there and available to us—however we do not have access to this until we turn on the light switch. We can optimize tapping and plugging into The Creator's light when we consciously choose to turn on The Creator's light switch; that is to say, when we choose to connect to our source, The Creator, thus receiving Its benefits.

The benefits of increasing your connection to The Creator includes:

- Raising your capacity to more fully tap into the light of The Creator.

- Enabling easier access to your bandwidth's wisdom and inner guidance.

- Increasing your alignment with The Creator, resulting in living life with more flow and ease and fulfilling your life purpose.

- Increasing capacity to experience Oneness Living.

- Expanding your love energy and radiance.

- Being more fully present in the now moment.

- Having more mental clarity.

When a person lives from ego/fear and in a more unconscious, unawaken state, their life tends to be more difficult. One reason for this is there is more mind chatter and therefore less ability to hear their inner guidance. Also, in this ego-driven state of being, they have a much greater tendency to perceive others as being separate from themselves. This often results in less awareness, or no awareness, of the unity of life.

Increasing one's connection to The Creator also commonly occurs through tragedy, pain, and intense difficulties in life. It is through this that a person can better understand the different aspects of themselves, especially when they are willing to explore, process, and learn from the painful experience. This can in turn cultivate a deeper and also better understanding of one's self, and can also support increased connection to The Creator.

EXERCISE

Here are two ways to increase your connection to The Creator:

Relax Your Mind

When your mind is in a more relaxed state through calming techniques like meditation, you have less mind chatter and can therefore better hear your inner guidance. It is as if the flower petals of a rose are prompted to open slowly, allowing more of what is inside to be seen. Through this, you cultivate the state of being awake and aware, along with increased mindfulness, naturally leading to hearing your inner wisdom, which supports greater connection with The Creator. You will also support an increased relaxed mind by pausing a few moments several times daily to consciously calm down during a busy day at work, for example.

Heart Space Living

As we have previously seen, living from your heart space increases your energetic vibration, love being the highest. This supports you becoming more aligned with The Creator, which naturally results in increased connection with The Creator.

You may want to read the exercises in Call Forth Love Through Your Heart Space chapter again on how to open your heart space.

Having an open heart is a lifeline to experience the unity of all life, which also supports connecting with The Creator.

Overcoming Difficulties

E ach of us have a defined path we must take. The journey of a thousand steps starts with the first one. In the defining moments of our lives we experience the necessary awakening that brings about change. In the same way the butterfly goes through the massive change in the cocoon, we too experience this. Often, this occurs through experiencing a difficult and painful physical disruption, such as a major injury or an illness.

There are various techniques and actions you can use to help you process trauma, pain, and other difficulties from physical injury or illness. The following is a partial list from many to consider. There are additional available modalities, including, of course, medical treatment that a person is using, as well as alternative treatment. Some people find it helpful to also include getting professional counseling or coaching to supplement their physical healing. Use your inner guidance system to help you choose. As always, offer yourself non-judgment, compassion, and kindness. You will also benefit by going into your heart space to raise your vibration as best as you can to invoke your love for your healing journey.

- Forgive yourself first. People tend to think they are at fault, when most of the time, it is not true.

- It is helpful to have someone in your life you can completely trust and rely on who will play a role of a sentinel and guide, and be an ever-abiding wall of strength for you. This person can help guide you with a loving approach.

- You are encouraged to explore within, and when ready and willing, to look boldly into this physical injury directly. Talk to that area of the body that has the injury or illness to find out what wisdom it has to share with you and what lesson there is for you to learn.

- Releasing your anger and frustration, or any other emotion, of the physical issue will help you gain peace within. Do this through healthy processing of the emotions, seeing a professional counselor, therapist, or trusted friend. Find an alternative and/or traditional healing modality may also support releasing emotions that need to be freed.

- Daily prayer to the injured part of the body, as well as talking to, and checking in with the area of the body that is injured. Offer gratitude for its dedication to supporting you.

- It will help you to be kind to it for this area of the body is an *extension of you*. In your awareness of treating this area kindly and with gratitude, you will also offer this to *yourself*. This will start the ball rolling for true healing. This will provide the solid foundation upon which your work on the *physical* plane will become effective, resolving the pain and also supporting an increased acceptance, *true acceptance*, of this whole injury or illness journey.

- When you come to full acceptance and gratitude and even love toward this physical area of your body, you will provide the rich fertilizer unto which true healing will occur. You will gain better clarity on what option or options to choose for the appropriate healing modalities to continue or to take up.

- You will find that going deep into contemplation and meditation for the purpose of deep cleansing, forgiving yourself, acceptance of the injured body part, and gratitude for this will facilitate even greater healing. This may lead to a whole new freedom, opening, expansiveness, less pain, and inner peace.

- Eating healthy foods and minimizing or eliminating unhealthy foods (such as sugar, gluten, dairy, processed foods, and acidic foods) will optimize feeling better and improve your immune system. Keeping your vibration high also greatly improves your immune system.

- Consciously taking care of your physical body is as important in maintaining your higher vibrations as when you do so through the mental and emotional techniques described earlier.

- Become aware of products you put into, or are considering to put into, your physical body, such as drugs or alcohol. In addition, be mindful of what someone else, such as a medical professional or friend, may suggest you use. Do a thorough research on that which you are considering to use. This way, you are well-informed on any side effects, along with benefits, of what goes into your physical body. Remember that you are the steward of your own body!

EXERCISE

Here is a loving and compassionate approach to dealing with your physical injury or illness. As with any exercise or healing modality, it is best you approach this with love in your heart, compassion for yourself, nonjudgment, and patience. Create a space where you feel safe and comfortable, and which offers you privacy. You may do this alone or with a trusted friend.

Compassionate Healing

Sit quietly with this area of your body, looking at it and *feeling* love and gratitude. Set an intention to hear what it has to share with you, without judgment. Be willing to listen to its words of wisdom, inviting it to share openly. You may want to grab a pen and paper and write down what you hear. You will do best to have an open heart while doing this.

Caress it and talk with it. Offer it, and yourself, love; through this, forgive yourself if you feel the need to do so. Allow the process to continue for as long as necessary, being patient and kind. Of course, ask for assistance from your angels, your friends, a counselor or coach, and from The Creator.

Light a candle, or do something else symbolic of the new path you will take to resolve the pain. Take a special token, memento, or rock to place with the candle. Invoke lots of love, gratitude, acceptance *into* this token. Take this token with you everywhere as a reminder of your new attitude/stance/perspective around your physical issue.

Set an intention to experience newness, new life, new energy, new capacity to feel and *be* healthier, and to indeed experience lasting relief for yourself and the injured area.

Let this intention of newness/revitalization through this meditation, contemplation, acceptance, gratitude, and love be the beacon of light to show you the way to the new that you *can* create for yourself.

Next, take the token you used with the candle and find a place to sit in nature. Stay here for as long as you would like, soaking in the new and refreshing energy you have created from this process. Now, intend for expansive inner peace and to have all the guidance and clarity on action steps to be taken to heal the injured area. Then pray and intend you *do* take those action steps as soon as feasible.

You can increase the probability of minimizing the physical issue or being free of it through your diligence, your self-love, self-acceptance, and self-forgiving!

When you can resolve the physical issue, not only are you supporting yourself, but you are also supporting humanity's positive change. How? By contributing peace and a sense of well-being to the collective consciousness.

Three Blessings for Daily Living

You can start each day by placing into your heart three blessings: blessing of the breath, blessing of life, and blessing of the Divine presence, which is always with you. When you wake up each morning, give great thanks for these three blessings. Be aware of them. Feel them. Cradle them. In doing so, you will feel love in your heart grow to big proportions. This is a wonderful way to set the tone for the day. You will also notice as you do this as a daily practice, your vibrational radiance and frequency increases. This results in a more stable vibratory resonance in your own field of life and beingness.

1. Blessing of the breath: Focus on the breath and know that the lungs already know how to automatically give you this life. Be keenly aware of your breath going in, then your breath going out. Offer gratitude for your lungs and the breath keeping you alive.

2. Blessing of life: For a few minutes, simply pay attention to and feel the universal life force energy

(chi) pulsating through you. Bathe in this sweet feeling, and remember each day is a gift of life.

3. Blessing of the Divine presence: Feel and connect to the Divine presence of life within you by centering yourself and by opening your heart. This supports increasing your vibration, which results in easier connection to The Creator. Hold dear to the knowing that this Divine presence always provides for you, offers you life, and allows you to have conscious awareness.

Complementary and Alternative Medicine (CAM)

There are many complementary and also alternative healing modalities that are available today, with a few of them listed below. As always, it is best when you follow your inner guidance to decide which CAM methods resonate with you, then research that, and once you have decided on the modality, find a reputable practitioner offering this. Many of the alternative healing modalities can be used also with traditional medical care you may currently be using. Feel free to check with your medical doctor on this as well as also checking with your intuition.

Acupuncture

Universal life force energy (chi) that is specific to the human body flows through meridians, which are certain pathways throughout the body. Acupuncture is a wholistic health technique for balancing our chi energy by inserting thin needles into specific points along these meridians.

This healing modality supports both physical as well as emotional well-being. It originated in China over 2,000 years ago from Traditional Chinese Medicine practices and is beneficial for relieving pain, removing energy blocks, and addressing various physical ailments. By having our chi energy flow more easily and properly, our bodies have an increased ability to heal itself.

Ayurvedic Medicine

Ayurveda is a whole-body approach to healing, believing there is a balance between the mind, body, and spirit. It is one of the oldest wholistic approaches to healing, developed in India about 3,000 years ago.

Rather than basing the healing approach through fighting a disease, Ayurveda focuses on promoting good health. Treatments of course can also be focused on a specific health issue as well as working proactively with maintaining good health.

This healing approach believes that everything is connected. When your mind, body, and spirit are in harmony with The Creator, then a person is in good health. Various conditions can disturb a person's proper balance and harmony, such as injuries, genetic or birth defects, seasonal changes, emotional upset, stress, and other factors. Illness can set in as a result.

Chiropractic Medicine

The area of focus and treatment of chiropractic medicine is on the relationship, and manual manipulation of, the skeleton, muscles, and nerves of a patient's body. Great emphasis is also placed on the spinal column in chiropractic treatments. Daniel David Palmer was the inventor of chiropractic in the late 1800s. He based his healing modality on his extensive anatomy and physiology studies as well as being quite prolific with studying many different areas of science.

It is also believed that having chiropractic adjustments improve the overall well-being and health of the patient and can support preserving and maintaining positive health. Treatments also have been found to relieve pain and discomfort a patient experiences when a part of their body is out of alignment. It is well known that everything in the physical body is connected and affected by other parts of the body, so when one area of the body is put back into alignment, other areas of the body benefit.

Emotional Freedom Technique (EFT)

EFT, also known as tapping, is based on the use of acupressure and acupuncture points on specific areas of the upper body. Tapping also draws on neurolinguistic programming, energy medicine, and Thought Field Therapy. Gary Craig is the originator of EFT. He graduated from Stanford, is a Certified Master Practitioner of Neuro Linguistic Programming and studied other forms of Energy Psychology.

Using your fingertips to tap on specific points, known as meridians (channels where chi flows) will stimulate those areas. This causes negative emotions to be released.

Homeopathy

Homeopathy is a medical system with the premise that our bodies can heal themselves by using natural products like plants and minerals. This modality was developed in Germany over 200 years ago, based on the methodology of treating disease with minute doses of a plant or mineral remedy and is recognized as an effective treatment.

This wholistic treatment is based on the individual, their symptoms and their history. It also addresses the emotional and mental aspects of the patient; therefore, along with helping to alleviate pain and address a physical illness, it also can help with, for example, anxiety and depression.

Ho'oponopono

Originating in Hawaii, Ho'oponopono is a powerful ancient prayer for reconciliation and forgiveness. The premise of this prayer is that when we ourselves take responsibility for what others are going through, not only can we heal ourselves, but we also heal others. This is because all life is connected. Hawaiian tradition believes in the interconnection as well.

A remarkable example of the success of this prayer was in 1984, with Dr. Hew Len, an expert on Ho'oponopono. He worked as a staff psychologist for a Hawaiian state hospital's ward for the out of control criminally insane. Previous attempts from other psychologists to resolve this were unsuccessful. After three years of Dr. Hew Len's work at this hospital, the ward for this group of patients was closed because all the patients improved and were healed! How did this happen? Dr. Hew Len spent time with each of the patient's files (not directly with them), using the Ho'oponopono prayer with each of them. Dr. Hew Len explained "I didn't heal them. I healed the part of myself that created them."

There are four phrases used in this prayer: I am sorry. Please forgive me. Thank you. I love you. These can be repeated several times as you feel is needed. When you focus on these phrases with sincerity, you will support self-healing and also healing in others. You can find yourself less anxious, less upset, and have increased calm and inner peace. There can also be improvement with, for example, a relationship with whom you did this prayer for. This prayer is also wonderful for the world. For example: I'm sorry. Please forgive me for whatever is going on inside of me that manifests as war. Thank you. I love you.

Iridology

Iridology is the healing modality of examining the eye for any discolorations and markings, which help to determine any potential problem with the body. The overall wellness of a person can be assessed by having an iridologist read the iris of the eye. The reason this assessment can be made is due to the iris' nerve endings being connected to the optic nerve, the base of the brain and all of the body's tissues. Different sectors of the iris correspond to a certain area of the body.

Dr. Ignatz Peczely, a Hungarian physician, invented Iridology around 1893. The iridology practitioner uses special equipment to assess a patient's iris and compares this to an iris eye chart. It is believed that the iris' nerve fibers respond to tissue in the body and for this reason the iris can be "read" to assess different areas of the body.

Naturopathic Medicine

Naturopathy is a wholistic approach to healing founded in 1896 by Benedict Lust based on nature cure and also hydrotherapy. This system of healing uses several natural healing methods to address the client's symptoms. This approach considers the mind, body, and spirit, not just the physical body. A Naturopathic doctor offers primary health care, treatment and also preventive care. This approach is from the perspective of using the healing power of nature, using the least invasive and least toxic therapies, and to trust the inherent wisdom that the body has to heal itself.

A naturopathic doctor looks at the root cause of the client's condition and treats that, rather than treating the disease and covering up the symptoms.

Neurolinguistics Programming (NLP)

With Neurolinguistics Programming, there is the belief that there is a connection between our language, our neurology, and our life experiences, which have been programmed by past situations and events. Dr. Richard Bandler and John Grinder created this modality the 1970s.

A trained NLP practitioner can assist their clients in changing limiting behavior by using certain techniques developed through this modality, such as eye and body movements, and language, which is believed to affect the brain's (neurological) functions. Using NLP techniques support the client with self-improvement and interpersonal communication, as well as changing (reprogramming) beliefs to those that serve the client in a more positive way.

Reflexology

Reflexology is a complementary health therapy that recognizes that the thousands of nerve endings in the foot and hand correspond to certain muscle groups and organs in the body. By massaging or applying pressure to specific points on the foot or hand, stress is reduced, healing in the corresponding part of the body can occur, and a sense of overall well-being can occur.

This therapy was used in ancient Egypt and India. It was in the 1900s that Dr. William Fitzgerald developed the Zone Therapy, from which Reflexology was developed by Eunice Ingham in the 1930s. She believed that any blocks or congestion in any part of the foot reflects a corresponding area in the body.

Reiki Energy Healing

Reiki is the Japanese word for universal (Rei) life force energy (ki). As you recall, this is also known as chi or prana. It was rediscovered in Japan by Dr. Mikao Usui in the late 1800s. We say "rediscovered" because throughout human history, gentle hands on and touch has been associated with comfort and healing. For example, what do we typically do when we have a headache or stomach pain? We put our hands on it.

Reiki increases vibration to the energy field of a person's energy centers (chakras) and aura, releases blocks in our chakras, helps a person relax and reduce stress, and increases the flow of chi energy throughout the body. It works on all levels of our being—physical, mental, emotional and spiritual. The Reiki practitioner is someone who has been attuned to the specific energy of Reiki and is a conduit of it. This alternative healing modality is a gentle hands-on (or hands-off) healing that allows the transference of chi to the client.

Sound Therapy

Sound therapy is a vibrational medicine based on psychology and neurology and the principle that everything is energy and in a continual vibrational state. Each part of your body has its own unique vibration, also known as resonance. When the resonance within a certain part of the body is out of balance, sound healing can help it get back to its natural state. It has been used since ancient times by many cultures, including Greece, India and Egypt.

The healing power of sound comes from a variety of sources, including the human voice (chanting, toning, mantras), tuning forks, sound baths, singing bowls, humming, drumming and other musical instruments. Benefits of sound therapy include emotional well-being, stress reduction, improved cognitive and motor functioning, pain management, alleviating sleep disorders, depression and anxiety, and helping with post-traumatic stress disorder (PTSD).

In India, chanting is widely practiced using the ancient Indian language called Sanskrit. Chanting with Sanskrit words helps clear a person's chakras and raises one's consciousness and vibration.

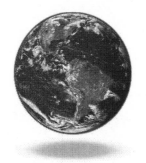

SECTION 4

Opportunities for Groups and Companies to Create Positive Change

Consider All Components

There is much discord on the planet today, as we are well aware. One of the largest components of creating peace once again is, as mentioned, to come into harmony with and in tune with the earth. We have spoken about the importance of offering love, kindness, and respect to one another, for this is a vital and large component of reestablishing peace on earth.

Another vital component is for people to be consistently aware of what action steps influence and impact the earth as well as her animals and all other life. It is best to consider all the possible consequences and impact of those action steps when a system is being developed.

For example, say there is a plan to develop a water treatment plant in a growing city. A new area of undeveloped land is being considered and this land is adjacent to a swamp area that houses a variety of animals and water life. In order to be respectful of, and live in harmony with, Mother Earth, it is critical to get environmental experts to properly establish the necessary criteria to create this water plant with minimal environmental impact. Future growth needs of this plant to accommodate the city's future growth also needs to be put into the equation. Environmental studies and predictions, and a trend analysis of the swamp and surrounding areas should be performed to estimate the future swamp boundaries.

Considering all angles and factors of this is a much more wholistic approach, a more "at one" approach, where all the elements in the system are being considered. There is a much higher opportunity for a successful outcome using a wholistic approach. The swamp will then continue to be without the water plant's influence and the water treatment facility will meet the city's water and recycling needs.

What about the farm lands being impacted by insecticides and pesticides? This has a huge impact on the soil's composition, which in turn affects the quality of the food vegetation that comes from farming there. The impact of these chemicals is such that the animals, birds, bees, and insects are negatively impacted, as evidenced by the growing number of bird species having a higher mortality rate of young newly hatched baby birds. The eggs' shells are thinner, offering a less than healthy embryonic environment for them. When there is less bird population to naturally eat the insects that infest the farmed produce, the increase in these insect populations stimulate the belief that more insecticides are needed for insect population control, when in fact a minimal amount of this insecticide application would be better. Let nature take its true course and let the birds eat the insects.

The impact of pesticides and insecticides also negatively affect the water quality of the water tables below and the runoff water. This in turn pollutes the water channeled to surrounding soil and any that ends up in a water treatment plant. Consideration of the level of concentration, quantity, and type of insecticides and pesticides should be carefully considered in order to apply this with the wholistic approach where *all* aspects of what will be impacted would be considered. Being in tune with, and awareness of, every aspect provides more respectful farming and cultivates a Oneness Living modality of life.

These chemicals, when ingested by people and animals, also has a negative influence on the body's functions. In time, when there is a cumulation of these chemicals in the body, disease may be created and the quality of life is impacted; animals exhibit similar symptoms of disease. When farming can be approached in a similar fashion as it had hundreds of years ago, before the onset of using chemicals, the quality of the soil, the birds, the animals, the people, and the water are healthier and better. Letting nature do what it does best— keeping the ecosystem in proper balance with its *natural* life forms—does yield a more optimal, respectful system. When artificial elements, such as insecticides and pesticides, are put into the ecosystem, there is a disruption of the natural flow of that ecosystem. Without the use of the chemicals, farm production can go back and resume its more in tune with nature approach and produce a better and healthier outcome.

Yes, some will argue that the use of insecticides has yielded more crops due to less insects, but what needs to be considered is the extent to which the elements within the ecosystem are being impacted by that. What is needed are more natural components to be used in making the insecticide solutions versus using chemicals. They can produce the same effect without the harsh chemicals.

This is also seen with household cleaners. Natural ingredient cleaners work just as well as harsh chemicals. The natural ingredients work more in harmony with nature; therefore, more in tune with and in sync with the ecosystem. There is a high negative impact to all of the elements involved— water, people, plants, animals—when harsh chemicals are used in the household.

Let us recognize the importance of approaching what we are doing within our own households or creating a new water treatment plant or applying optimal farming methods; that when considering how *all* elements within the system gets impacted, this wholistic, respectful, and mindful approach offers the proper consideration for Mother Earth. This in turn has a domino effect of impacting our own lives.

Can you imagine what it would be like when the majority of businesses and households worldwide are in harmony with the earth?

Ingredients Needed to Create an Optimal Outcome

There are particular circumstances that yield particular kinds of crops and the amount of harvest that comes with it. When there is consistent rain, the crop's yield tends to be maximized, and when the rain is not consistent, the yield will be less. There is a greater opportunity to have a positive outcome when we, as humanity, can be consistent with our exposure to, and our offering of love and respect; the propensity is a higher yield to create more peace on earth. When there is turmoil and discord among the masses, more often than not, the propensity to yield a higher level of peace drops dramatically. The momentum of resources needed to create peace is squelched. The proper level of required ingredients is necessary to yield the desired outcomes. By assessing what is necessary to create the desired outcome, we can better facilitate that outcome.

The same is true with the planning and the organization involved when creating a desired outcome through any type of system, an event or a business, for example. What are the strategic components needed to get from here to there? How is this accomplished most efficiently? What components outside of the planned system need to be considered to minimize a negative impact? Are there resources available that will maximize the desired outcome most effectively? In what ways can the event be promoted to maximize the outcome? There are ways to approach creating an event or a business that optimize the circumstances to create more harmony, efficiency, and to promote consideration of all components effected. When you also consider the external factors on your decision-making process, you can create a more favorable outcome.

When *all* systems are considered, including assessing what components of each of those systems are involved, there will be a higher opportunity to experience more efficiency, cooperation, and consideration for *all* concerned.

The same is true with humanity's state of affairs. We can maximize the state of peace by using the right ingredients. To do so requires retraining of the mind. One major way to create peace is through teaching people about Oneness Living. Respect, kindness, harmony, love, and support for ourselves and for others and the planet are some of the ingredients necessary to cultivate the Oneness Living perspective with increased effectiveness and efficiency. In the same manner that the apple tree yields more apples when given the right amount of water and other environmental conditions, when the planet and humanity are given the right ingredients the outcome naturally yields a higher amount of peace on the planet.

Of course, the question is, how do we get there? We get there by starting with you! When you work on increasing your self-love, respect, kindness, harmony, cooperation, and support, you are not only benefiting yourself but also those around you and equally humanity since each of us contribute to the collective consciousness. This is a great way you can help change humanity's current state of affairs. Living from these higher vibrations offers an increased amount of the necessary ingredients to create increased peace on earth.

Likewise, when a corporation or other type of organization focuses on considering *all* necessary ingredients in their strategic planning and also in their creating a new system or process, then there can be an increased efficiency, harmony, respect, kindness, cooperation, and support throughout.

Actions That Groups Can Take

A s you have read, there are many actions you, as an individual, can take, such as using the exercises shared here in this book. As you know, taking action creates positive change and transformation within your own life and those around you as well as contributing to humanity's collective consciousness.

You may also want to take additional action through any of the following group activities listed below, or other group activities found elsewhere. If so, you are encouraged to explore these and to empower yourself to step up and get active with that group!

Keep in mind, when being involved with any type of group activity that it is best to be well-informed on the issues that any other party on that same issue has. To better facilitate your group's increased understanding of their perspective, be with an open heart and open mind to what their viewpoint is. To assist in this, get yourself and your group into increased energetic vibration (if not already there), to ensure all participants of your group are coming from love instead of fear. Also, set a positive environment for optimal nonviolent communication by setting an intention that both sides have an open heart and open mind to sincerely hear what the other party has to say, and use any applicable exercises to facilitate that state of being. Cultivate having respect, love, kindness, cooperation, and peace for all parties involved, so that energetically and on the physical level, a more harmonious outcome is achieved.

Activism

Is there a cause that you are passionate about? Would you like to advocate for this cause? Perhaps it is for better treatment of the environment or to help eradicate child trafficking or to keep the right of choosing what goes into your body or what does *not* go into your body.

Whatever the cause may be, if you want your voice heard and to also inform people on facts of the particular cause you support, consider taking the stand by becoming an activist. Activism involves using direct action to either support or to be against a particular issue or cause. The purpose of this is to facilitate achieving a particular goal for a political or social change. Writing a letter to a government representative, attending a peaceful march or demonstration, having discussions in small groups, boycotting something or volunteering for a group or nonprofit are some examples of activism.

You can become a member of a coalition, activist or advocacy group or other cohorts that support the same cause you are passionate about. When enough people join together, this forms an even more powerful synergy of energy than if only one person does it alone. Remember, we are social beings with the innate need to be in community. Working together by taking action and creating heightened awareness of *all* issues involved with a cause is a powerful way to facilitate social and political change.

Lobbying

Lobbying can be a paid or unpaid activity that informs our government representatives pertinent information regarding specific legislation to help them be more informed with their decision making. With the United States constitution, we have the right to lobby.

Here are two actions you may want to consider regarding lobbying, either on your own, or even better, with a coalition or advocacy group:

- Attend a committee hearing on a particular piece of legislation you want to be part of and either testify or be an observer.

- Go to the House and to the Senate's gallery area and submit the required paper requesting to see a particular Representative or Senator in person (check your local government for the dates they have this). If the Representative or Senator is available at that time, they will come out to talk directly to you, which at that time you can succinctly share the points regarding the legislation you want to inform them about.

Asset-Based Community Development (ABCD)

ABCD is an approach to solving problems within a community that is based on focusing on what the community's strengths are, instead of focusing on what their deficits are. Focusing on their strengths is empowering because it looks at the community problems as being solved by using the community's assets (gifts and strengths the individuals and the community have).

In this model, community members are seen as part of the solution rather than merely recipients of support from outside agencies such as government or nonprofits. This model provides a methodology for developing communities in a sustainable manner and includes community members in the decision making of solving problems. This increases their involvement in their own community and provides an impetus to continue being involved.

ABCD was developed by John L. McKnight and John P. Kretzmann at the Institute for Policy Research. They published a book in 1993 called *Building Communities from the Inside Out: A Path Toward Finding and Mobilizing A Community's Assets.*

Indeed, as you have just read, this ABCD model is used for communities. Let us use our imagination to think about what it would be like if the company you work for took the ABCD's approach of recognizing your strengths and is sincerely willing to consider what you have to say regarding a particular issue at work. What would it be like when all employees were equally included in any decision-making process that involves them directly? How empowered do you think your coworkers and yourself would feel? In what way would you behave differently working for a company that hears what you have to say and takes that into consideration with their decision making? It would be supportive for the planet when more companies worldwide took the stance of recognizing their employees' strengths and including them in their decision-making processes.

Diversity, Equity and Inclusion

Fortunately, there is a growing trend for companies and other organizations to include the concept of Diversity, Equity and Inclusion (DE&I) into their policies. There are many definitions for DE&I. It can generally be said that DE&I is the attempt to being more welcoming to the diverse types of people in any organization, along with recognizing the need to treat people with more equity and inclusion within the institution or company.

Diversity includes all the ways in which people are different and recognizing that some people will identify with multiple identities. These identities include ethnicity, color, race, sexual orientation, marital status, nationality, religion, socioeconomic status, veteran status, education level, language, age, gender and gender expression, as well as mental or physical abilities and learning.

People often ask what the difference is between equity and equality. Equality is when there is equal opportunity given for all populations of a society, whereas equity offers varying levels of resources and support, depending on the need, to *achieve fairness of outcomes across the board.* Certain populations may have certain barriers and therefore require additional resources and support to *bring them to the same level* as other populations.

Inclusion promotes offering sincere respect and support to *everyone* in the organization and making them feel important and included. Inclusion also allows for all people in the organization to participate fully in any decision-making processes and provide opportunities across the board. This is similar to the model that ABCD offers, as we have just seen.

An important component of inclusion also includes recognizing and addressing unconscious biases that many people have through training employees and implementing company policies.

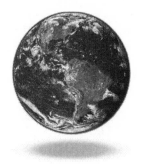

SECTION 5

In Conclusion

Birthing the New Earth

Each of us, in our own way bring about change, for within each of us are the seeds of change. As with the changing times on our dear Mother Earth, so too is humanity changing. As we have seen, change is necessary to bring about the new earth. Oneness Living, harmony, kindness, respect, love, and peace, which represent some of the characteristics of this new earth, can only come into full fruition when each of us, as well as corporations, governments, and other organizations, contributes positively to the much-desired new earth.

In these ever-changing times, now more than ever, you are being called to awaken from your dream of separation, walk your authentic life and come to a deeper fulfilment of your true path in life; that of true peace, love, respect, kindness, and harmony within yourself, with others around you, with your community, and with Mother Earth. You can start by understanding that you are one with The Creator. Realizing this will help you to live more in alignment with who you really are, a divine being made in the image of The Creator. Also recognize that everyone else is also made in the image of The Creator. This is one of the critical and effective ways to support the necessary transformation in humanity to having a new earth and an improved, optimal way of living.

As you know by now, each of us, along with businesses and other organizations, contribute to the vibration of the planetary ecosystem and collective consciousness through our unique vibrational essence and signature. Through this, we *collectively* synthesize those vibrational energies. So why not consciously create the collective combined energies to be of higher vibration, which is necessary to bring about a greater momentum of the peace we desire to experience?

There are still many people who are resisting and putting negative energy out, attempting to maintain the old earth's patriarchal and competitive ways of living. Fortunately, the grip of the ego's stronghold of this way of living is beginning to loosen up due to the old patriarchal and competitive ways no longer fitting in with the new vibration/fabric/makeup of the new earth that is forming. The resistance and negative energy of the old ways results in the rubbing up against the new earth's fabric, causing what we witness as the natural outcome of increased discord, violence, unrest, and worldwide disharmony.

The people who do not process and let go of their pain and upsets will continue to struggle and contribute lower vibrational energies to the collective whole. But as more people find the way to better living, that is, to ascend and awake, the more light and higher vibration is contributed to the planet. This then offsets the lower vibrations, supporting humanity's ascension to the new earth.

What are we to do? There are some people who feel their fabric of life is deteriorating and they do not know what to hold on to. It is as if the world is crumbling and there is nothing to stand on. They may feel dismayed, unsettled, apprehensive, fearful, hopeless, angry. The remedy lies in the knowing to stand in faith. In this manner, a new foundation is built. How does one build this new foundation of faith? By being in alignment with your true self, which is the same thing as saying being in alignment with The Creator, the divine source of all.

To be in alignment with your true self means to live your life from the true essence of you by experiencing higher vibrations of the positive emotions such as love, harmony, gratitude, and kindness, which in turn brings you happiness and inner peace. Experiencing life this way allows you to more fully live in tandem with The Creator, the source which gives you life.

How do you live with alignment to your true self, thus creating a new foundation of faith? Here are some actions you can take, some which have already been shared and worth repeating:

- Meditating will assist you with connecting more with The Creator.

- Process through and heal the old ways that do not serve you so you can release and let them go. You can gain hope by knowing that as the old ways release, new positive ways are being formed.

- Knowing deeply—with full faith—that all you
  require to live is provided for you and that you are
  never alone. You can relax more with life this way.

- Keep your chi/life energies flowing by keeping your
  heart open, be in the space of love, and do chi
  conditioning exercise and practices.

This new way, the new earth, *is* the new foundation. It *will* be created, and in fact is in the midst now of being created, whether a person actively participates in the process or not. However, if unaware and not actively participating, life becomes more of a struggle. Why? Because it takes a lot of energy to fight and resist it. Many people continue to live this way, creating continued discord within themselves, which as we know, also impacts others and the collective consciousness.

We can make the "birthing process" into this new earth easier by allowing the process to happen and to take an active part in creating our improved individual lives as well as contributing to the new earth.

In addition to the suggested actions just shared, here are other actions you can take, some which we have covered earlier:

- Live consciously by examining your old ways,
  beliefs and patterns that do not serve you. Then
  be willing to dismantle, process through and then
  release these instead of holding onto them. You

may or may not need to get professional support with this.

- Rewire your neuro pathways by repeatedly and consistently thinking positive and loving thoughts, saying uplifting and kind words, and acting in higher vibrational ways.

- Be more positive and more from the place of alignment with The Creator. This will help you better maintain a higher vibrational state and will help maintain longer periods of times of higher love energy, increased harmony, and peaceful vibrations. This leads to you being able to better connect with The Creator.

- Be willing to own not only those personality traits you like about yourself, but also those you do *not* like. Each of us have aspects that we bury deep within because we cannot face them or admit we have these. Yet when you can own *all* aspects of yourself, you are more fully accepting yourself, resulting in feeling better about yourself as well as others. Why? Because, as you will recall, what you see in others is a reflection of what is actually also in you! Know you are safe to accept *all* of who you are. Be willing to process and release any shame or dislike you may have around your disowned personality traits. You can also use this as an impetus to make positive change with yourself.

Similarly, when you realize your own gifts and talents, you naturally have more of the ability to see the gifts and talents in others, again due to our outpicturing of that which is inside of us.

- Find the good in yourself so you can increase your self-esteem and confidence. Through this, you cultivate the inherent positive qualities that only you can offer the world through your unique combinations of traits.

- Nurture and cultivate more self-love. This results in you feeling better about yourself and you are also better able to share your gifts and talents with others as well as give more love.

- Consciously be aware of how you treat your physical body by being an excellent steward of it. Just as it is vital to properly care for your emotional, mental, and spiritual bodies, you will feel better and increase your vibration when taking positive care of your physical body. This includes being mindful of *everything* you put into your body—and also that which you do not want to put into your body— such as the food you eat, any medications or supplements, alcohol and any other type of product that your body has to process. The higher your vibration, the higher your immune system will be, which of course supports your overall wellbeing.

- Be environmentally friendly in ways that still support your lifestyle and also respects our Mother Earth. Here are some (of many) simple actions you can incorporate into your daily life:

  - Recycle as much as possible.

  - Bike to work or take public transportation once or more each week.

  - Save water
    - Turn off the water while brushing your teeth, washing your hands, and while handwashing dishes, then turn it back on to rinse.
    - Avoid cleaning your driveway with water. Use a broom instead.
    - Minimize eating meat. Several research studies have shown it takes anywhere from 1,590 to 2,000 gallons of water to produce one pound of beef! Most water usage is from feed production and meat processing.

- Minimize paper use by:
  - Paying your monthly bills online instead of using paper invoices.
  - Use recycled paper.
  - Minimize using paper napkins and paper towels. Use cloth instead.

- o When possible, use hemp and bamboo products instead of products made from trees.
- Minimize using plastic by:
  - o Reuse plastic as much as you can, such as plastic sandwich bags and grocery bags. Better yet, use canvas grocery bags.
  - o Use refillable water bottles instead of one-time use plastic water bottles.
  - o When available, purchase products with minimal amount of packaging.
- If you are in a management position and/or own your own business, make conscious decisions for new or existing projects, products, procedures, and systems by considering what the highest and best good will be for all employees, clients, the environment, the organization, and any other system components.

You are here to examine, learn, and to create healing with yourself and the planet, and to create a new way of being. When you do this, you contribute to the much-needed change that humanity is crying for!

The time has come to step into the new arena of the new earth. You can facilitate this process by doing your own work. Not only do you benefit, but those around you benefit, and indeed, the planet as a whole will benefit as well.

A Call to Action

The time to act is now! The time has come for everyone on earth to unite to create change. In the whole scheme of things, we are but a drop in the vast ocean of eternal life. But we each are here now, experiencing the wide array of human emotions, from pain and hatred, all the way to the other extreme of compassion and love. We are of the human race; yes, however, we are of The Creator! Each one of us are, in our birthright, the divine essence. The very makeup of who we are defines us as sacred. Divine. Worthy. Deserving in every way of living life in a happy, fulfilling, loving, peaceful way.

There are some who believe the time has come for the second coming of Christ. This theology gives hope for a new earth, yes, however, another way to look at this is that the second coming of Christ is the rebirth and the awakening of each person to Oneness Living. To living life from higher vibrational emotions. To respect and honor all life and Mother Earth. To view life as sacred. To hold the flower in your hand seeing the beauty of The Creator in it. To hear the cry of a newborn baby's new life. To witness the sacred passage into womanhood, the profound mighty oak tree in the forest, the birds chirping, welcoming spring time once again. The twinkling stars, the shining moon, the life-giving warmth of the sun. To all this, who do we give thanks? To the all-encompassing, loving Creator of course. Include also the remembrance that all this, and more, is an intricate and integral part of the whole, of The Creator.

Yes, there is the upset, war, hatred, misunderstandings between people and between nations. Yet with all of this so prevalent, there is also the ever-increasing compassion, kindness, and service offered for the improvement of humanity: the outpouring of love and also monetary support to natural disaster victims, the continuous generous giving to the millions of starving people, the positive work done by environmentalists, the dedication of those involved with activism, the many nonprofits offering to improve life for the homeless and others in need, the everyday heroes working endlessly to provide care for the sick, the underserved, the animals. There are many more examples of the widespread good continuously being poured forth in droves, despite the few that are continuing to attempt to grow their machine of greed and power.

In the end, it all comes down to the masses having the final say—we are here to uphold the good in others. We are here to serve for the betterment of all humanity. We are here offering kindness to our neighbors, support to the underserved and marginalized populations, advocacy for the underprivileged. We are here to unite together to propagate what we desire (unconsciously or consciously)—the new earth.

Together, with more people awakening, we will prevail! We will remain strong in our conviction that Oneness Living, goodness, kindness, and respect for *all* life is the optimal way of living! We will combine our efforts to stand up to corruption, power, and greed of the few. We will prevail. We will succeed. We are one united! In doing this, the future of humanity has hope for a better earth, where we walk unencumbered, free from strife, war, and famine. For through change, comes transformation. This transformation is the Age of Aquarius, the new earth, the new template of life called love and peace.

So be encouraged with this infusion of hope and clarity. You are asked to carry forth your part of the implementation of humanity's cry for change. When many of us take action for transformative change, the Hundredth Monkey Effect will occur, thus the shift to this new way of living will take place.

Bringing It All Together

In an effort to bring it all together, think of a time you have been in a special place that brings you joy and pleasure. It could be a beautiful lake, meadow, or an ocean view. Imagine yourself being here in this special place and hold the space in your heart. Sit with the feeling and memory of this place. Quieting the mind, now imagine in this place a gathering of many people throughout the land, coming together also feeling calm, joyful, and quiet. You see off in the distance there are many others coming toward this large open special place joining you and the others already here. They are also peaceful, happy, and content.

As more people gather into this big area of open space, each one in their own blissful, relaxed state of being, there is a drum roll in the center of this open space. You see the drummer sitting at a large Native American Indian drum, one that sits on the floor and is very wide and large. This lone drummer is beating the drum in a wonderfully rhythmic beat, and as the drummer continues to drum in this fashion, more are answering the call of the drumming.

What this drumming and the gathering represents are the continual increase of people hearing the call of humanity's cry for change. They are choosing to answer this call! The call that we are in the very midst of; the current paradigm shift in which the changes of the planet, and with each one of us, are being lovingly asked to answer and fulfill. *This is the call of humanity to wake up* and to take the invitation of joining the many others who have already answered the call. By answering this clarion call, each one of us contributes to their own inner shift, which naturally contributes to the collective consciousness' shift.

Look into the eyes of your brothers and sisters, and you are also looking into the eyes of yourself. We are all one united together bringing forth the expression of The Creator here on earth.

In this gathering of so many people, there is the unification and synergistic culmination of an even higher level of perspective and knowing within each person, and as a community, called humanity. It is the knowing that as we, humanity, gather and join, we are combining our efforts of creating and helping the birthing process. The birthing of the new earth, along with the birthing of each individual who cares to join in.

For those who are not quite ready, or for those who are still in the throes of their pain, this gathering, the collective synergy of the elevated vibration, upholds and nurtures them. For when there are enough people in this gathering, it supports tipping the scales, that is, creating enough of a momentum to hold up the light and love for those who are still in the disillusionment of the lower vibrations and pain. The light that has formed as a result of all these people gathering, and the concurrent benefit to the planet, creates a sweet, quiet stillness. Pause now to feel this sweet silence.

In this stillness there is the joy and deep experience of peace. A sweet knowing that we have reached the required level of consciousness that carries humanity, as a dove carries the olive branch to the levels of love, the highest universal vibration. In this is the seed of everlasting peace on this dear Mother Earth.

Imagine with me the knowing you would have in your heart of this peace, this joy, and this love. It is the representation of the new earth's paradigm. Will you now join me in holding this vision for yourself, for your children and your children's children, and all of humanity, knowing we are here joining with Mother Earth in peaceful unity?

The time has come. And it is now! Not one year or five years from now, but now. Feel the shift and change in your beingness, listen to your own heart's calling, and you will know when the right time will be to join that drum beat that is calling you! It is possible, it is happening. Now is the time to gather!

This offers you the hope so you can indeed heed humanity's call to rise above the current state of affairs of violence, war, disharmony, and self-hatred. And to bestow upon the earth the love and respect she deserves. In doing so, all of her inhabitants will be provided for with the healthy food and water necessary for survival, and the associated love, respect and kindness all life forms deserve.

Hear the drum beat. Listen to your heart and to your inner voice and take positive action. The urgent clarion call is here now for you to join.

Recommended Reading

A New Earth – Awakening to Your Life's Purpose,
by Eckhart Tolle

Asset Based Community Development, by Mike Green,
with Henry Moore and John O'Brien

Becoming Supernatural – How Common People are Doing the Uncommon, by Dr. Joe Dispenza

Evolve Your Brain – The Science of Changing Your Mind,
by Dr. Joe Dispenza

Fractal Time, by Gregg Braden

Letting Go, by David Hawkins, M.D., Ph.D.

Nonviolent Communication – A Language of Life,
by Marshall B. Rosenberg, Ph.D.

Radical Authenticity – Strong Medicine for Turbulent Times,
by David Steele

Sacred Quantum Metaphysics, by Rich Haas

The Astonishing Power of Emotions, by Esther and Jerry
Hicks, (The Teachings of Abraham)

The Divine Matrix, by Gregg Braden

The Dark Side of the Light Chasers – Reclaiming Your Power, Creativity, Brilliance, and Dreams, by Debbie Ford

The Field – The Quest for the Secret Force of the Universe, by Lynne McTaggart

The Four Agreements – A Practical Guide to Personal Freedom, by Don Miguel Ruiz

The Power of Intention – Learning to Co-create Your World Your Way, by Dr. Wayne W. Dyer

The Power of Now, by Eckhart Tolle

The Untethered Soul: The Journey Beyond Yourself, by Michael A. Singer

Acknowledgments

It is with immense honor and joy that I am able to share the vital teachings of this book. It is through the inspiration I receive while meditating that provides the wisdom found in these pages. It is with the deepest heartfelt gratitude that I thank The Creator for the loving insights I received for this book, my previous book, as well as what I receive in my daily life.

What a team of experts I have the privilege to work with! My deep gratitude to my editor Karen Reddick of The Red Pen Editor. Her book industry knowledge, honest opinions, as well as editing expertise is much appreciated. A big shout out to my creative graphic design artist, Natasha Brown, for the book cover design. With her broad range of skills, she was able to quickly assess how best to depict this book's message. I am grateful for the creativity and professionalism of Nick Zelinger. His attention to detail while formatting the layout of this book took the interior pages to the next level.

I appreciate the continuous support from my two children, Evan and Jamie, and am grateful in many ways for both of you being in my life. I also acknowledge my friends (you know who you are!) who are always there for me, offering your deep wisdom and unwavering support in all that I do and all that I am. I am so appreciative for the unconditional acceptance that is given to me by all my family members, both here in the states as well as abroad. My heartfelt appreciation for each of my Joyful Journey Sister Goddesses, for the supportive anchor so freely shared.

To the dance leaders of the Dances of Universal Peace community that I am active with: Bernie Heideman, Sky Roshay, Jennifer Friedman, Mary Ellen Garrett and Timothy Dobson. Each of you inspire and support *so many* in our community through your unwavering commitment to worldwide love and peace. For me, you each uplift and sustain my spirit and soul, allowing me to be rejuvenated so I may continue my work for humanity.

There are many lightworkers and awakened ones all across the globe, who continuously contribute their talents and love towards creating a better world. My heartfelt gratitude for your most important work and dedication.

My expansive and deep gratitude to you, my readers. You are an important piece of the puzzle in this experience called *Humanity's Cry for Change*. Thank you for stepping up and doing the work to heal yourself and heal the world. You are to be commended for your courage and strength!

About the Author

Kate Heartsong is an author, speaker, entrepreneur, coach, and Reiki Master/Teacher. The deep wisdom Kate shares comes from her unique gift of channeling profound wisdom while meditating, as well as the understanding she gained from overcoming her life's challenges, and insights she received from her transformation of self-discovery, resulting in finding her own voice, becoming empowered, and living authentically.

Since childhood she had dreamt of making the world a better place for all. It is not surprising she has received the inner guidance that has created this book *Humanity's Cry for Change!*

This journey Kate has taken provides the expansive passion, dedication, and compassion she has to serve her readers, clients, audiences, humanity, and Mother Earth.

Kate has the heart of a true humanitarian. For over 20 years she has been an active member of the Dances of Universal Peace community, promoting kindness, understanding, love, and respect through this and other communities. She is also a visionary leader, for it is her knowing that when we start with one person at a time, a ripple effect occurs supporting peace on a global level, because we are all interconnected. Kate's own inspirational quote says it best: "Peace within, peace on earth."

If you enjoyed this book, please write a review on Amazon.

This will help get the word out to support others and to create a new earth! Thanks!

To hire Kate to speak at your event, offer empowering workshops, or to have a one-on-one coaching session with her, contact her at *JoyfulRadiance.com.*

Made in the USA
San Bernardino, CA
15 July 2020

75338037R00141